Beyond the Lagoon

Beyond the Lagoon

Hoverdoctors to Papua New Guinea

CECIL D. PEARSE

HODDER & STOUGHTON AUSTRALIA
A member of the Hodder Headline Group

DEDICATION

To my dear wife Kath, without whose help and loving support none of this would have been possible for me.

To my children, Martin and Christine, who tackled the daunting task of telling their father it wasn't good enough and with whose help I hope it has been improved.

First published in 1993
by Hodder & Stoughton (Australia) Pty Limited
(A division of Hodder Headline)
10-16 South Street, Rydalmere, NSW, 2116.

ISBN 0 340 59941 3

Production and design by Modern Times Pty Ltd
Printed and bound in Great Britain by
Butler & Tanner Ltd, Frome and London

Contents

Acknowledgments

A book of this nature cannot be written without the help of many people and I want to thank all those who have played a part in helping me to complete it. First the members of the team whose story it is and who have willingly placed their trust in me; they have helped by giving me suggestions, notes and information without which the account would have been sparse and I am grateful to each of them for that, and for so readily providing the characters in our tales. I want also to thank all the folk at Balimo, Mapodo and in Port Moresby who showed such kindness to us during our stay there and who have too, in one way and another, provided me with much material.

I cannot say a big enough thank you to my family who have borne the brunt of my total absorption in the book for several months and my consequent neglect of them and of many other things during that time. Not only that but Kath, Christine and Martin have all played a part in encouraging me and in helping to improve my first laboured efforts. Martin, in particular, has worked hard to guide me, firmly resisting all pressures when he believed improvement was necessary and ruthlessly wielding an incisive editorial mind and pen to, I trust, good effect. My colleagues, too, have tolerated my distraction with an easy grace and I am grateful for that. I also want to thank Bert Hingley at Hodders for his help and encouragement. Working with an unknown author at a distance of many thousands of miles cannot be easy and yet he made it a painless process for me.

Finally Mike Cole, too, must feature here for without his efforts and vision the expedition would never have come into being. He it was who involved me in the first place and gave me the opportunity to take part in the expedition. I am grateful to him for that and for the confidence he placed in me by making me the official scribe.

Thanks to the efforts and help of all these people I have enjoyed working on the book. I can only hope that you, the reader, might enjoy the story too.

Foreword

As Patron of the expedition I was delighted to be asked to write a few words by way of an introduction to this fascinating book. The expedition, the fourth of its kind to be organised by Squadron Leader Michael Cole, has proved to be a fitting sequel to the achievements of its predecessors.

Beyond the Lagoon gives a remarkable insight into the severe problems that face the medical services in Papua New Guinea and the way in which the Hovercraft Expedition has overcome many of these difficulties in some of the remote rural areas.

The team comprising a group of individuals brought together by their Christian faith, faced many challenges during the three month expedition. Their story, told by Cecil Pearse, gives us a taste of the hardships they endured, the obstacles they overcame and the tremendous sense of achievement as their mission was accomplished.

Their faith clearly helped them to persevere against the odds and their endeavours will have given those they went to help a real foundation for the future.

It is a great honour for me to have been associated with both the project and the book and I am grateful to Cecil Pearse for allowing us to share their experiences.

Sir Edward Heath, KG, PC, MBE, MP

Preface

I first heard of the Hoverdoctors Expedition to Papua New Guinea from Sir Edward Heath, who as Patron of the expedition, invited my support in late 1992. Although I had not at that time visited Western Province, that part of Papua New Guinea in which Balimo, the site of the expedition, is situated, I knew from my travels elsewhere in the country that the communities living in such remote areas desperately need the kind of help which the Hoverdoctor Expedition offered. I had no hesitation in agreeing to help in any way possible.

I did wonder at the time about the timetable for the expedition sketched out by Sir Edward, for it seemed ambitious. Not only were there formidable problems involved in transporting such a novel form of transport (for Papua New Guinea) to contend with. Administrative and other pitfalls loomed. The Papua New Guinea Government had embarked on a wide ranging and quite radical programme of reform. Among other things, this had led to the suspension of the Western Province Provincial Government, which could have complicated the undertaking. Another potentially worrying development has been the introduction of a more rigorous regime for foreign medical personnel working in Papua New Guinea.

I need not have been so apprehensive. The Expedition already had an excellent support team in Port Moresby and Balimo and I later learned that they had already accomplished much to ensure success. Government Ministers, including the Prime Minister, and the Minister for Health the Hon. Francis Koimanrea, were particularly helpful. He later visited the United Kingdom as the guest of our Government and met Sir Edward Heath to discuss the progress of the expedition.

In the event, the timetable was respected and, as will be evident from Cecil Pearse's admirable account of the enterprise, Hoverdoctor's objective in helping to bring medical care to the people in the Balimo District was achieved. To those of us who travelled to Balimo from Port Moresby for the formal inauguration early in May 1993, the expedition had seemed a remarkably smooth operation, apparently untroubled by problems along the way. We did not suspect the extent to which the expedition members and their support team had been pushed in overcoming numerous obstacles which had threatened to seriously delay the project and, just occasionally, possibly render it nugatory. But teamwork, ingenuity and sheer determination won the day. Papua New Guinea needs more such initiatives. Already, the Hoverdoctor Expedition has aroused interest elsewhere in Papua New Guinea where isolated and poorly served communities could benefit from the kind of service now in place at Balimo. This is a wonderfully heartwarming tribute to the generosity of all those who gave — materially and spiritually — to ensure the success of the Balimo expedition.

J. W. Guy
High Commissioner
Port Moresby

Prologue

The snakebite need not have killed Maidame Kukupi. He was nine years old, fit and healthy. The hospital was only twelve miles (twenty kilometres) away at Balimo and there was a VHF radio link. The doctors there were good and they had anti-snakebite serum. Yet still Maidame Kukupi died, and he died in agony.

Maidame Kukupi's death resulted from circumstances common in remote areas of the undeveloped world. Medical services, if they exist, are often provided by an overstretched and underfunded mission hospital or aid post. Staff struggle valiantly to bring comfort and healing to as many as they can, yet the nature of the terrain and the lack of adequate transport limit the number they can reach easily or quickly. If available, air transport is expensive even when operated by charitable organisations such as the Mission Aviation Fellowship. Extensive road systems linking small, scattered communities are beyond the resources of the poorer countries. The few roads that do exist can become impassable even to tractors. In the wet season at Balimo it is not unknown for patients, flown in as emergency cases, to have to be carried on a stretcher as far as two and a half miles (four kilometres) through mud impassable to vehicles. Where rivers can be used for cheaper transport, travel can be slow and at the mercy of many delays. People suffer needlessly, and some die.

Papua New Guinea, where Maidame Kukupi lived, is the second largest island in the world, one-tenth the size of Australia. Maidame's home was in the remote tropical Fly River area, twenty million acres (eight million hectares) of swampland, the largest remaining in the world. The Aramia River, by which Maidame lived, is part of a vast network of swamps and lagoons. In this convoluted maze of interconnecting waterways, short and direct line-of-sight distances can take an age to cover. Water levels vary by as much as thirty feet (nine metres) between the wet and dry seasons. Massive monsoon floods race down from the mountains, bringing thousands of tonnes of silt into the delta area and changing the pattern of the channels and mudbanks. Dry seasons expose large areas of swampy shallows or mud, both of which are impassable; the mud is too thick for boat or canoe and too deep to wade through. When water levels are higher, floating water weed or tough grasses grow rapidly, cutting off whole communities. In the heat and high humidity of an area only eight degrees south of the equator, travel can be laboriously slow.

Exposed to moisture-laden winds for ten months of the year, New Guinea is one of the largest constantly wet areas in the world. It is also one of the wildest. Rainfall is often up to 160 inches (400 centimetres) a year, even as high as 280 inches (700 centimetres) in places, with temperatures in the ninety degree Fahrenheit (thirty degree Celcius) range and above. In the Fly region the diet comprises mainly sago meal, with perhaps coconut or fish. Successful hunters can add wallaby, cassowary or wild pig to relieve the monotony of the sago diet and, despite poor soil, a little attention to gardening can produce pumpkin or banana. With moderate effort, food is there to be gathered and malnutrition is not common. But there are hazards such as poisonous snakes, endemic malaria and the few remaining crocodiles. And if serious illness or injury strikes, as with Maidame Kukupi, it may not be possible to get the necessary help in time. Without on-the-spot medical help and antivenene the speed of a plane alone was not sufficient to save Maidame. A simple, rapid, readily available, and inexpensive means of transporting medical help was needed.

These are the day-to-day realities of life for the Gogodalas, a tribal group in the region of the Aramia and Fly rivers, one of a thousand tribes living mainly in remote rural areas of Papua New Guinea and between them speaking more than 700 distinct languages. Despite the difficulties and restricted resources the Balimo Health Centre provides a medical and primary health care service to the Gogodala and to a number of other tribes on the fringes of their area.

The doctors at Balimo wanted to overcome their transport difficulties. Hovercraft, they realised, could be the answer. A diverse group of people, gathered together by Mike Cole and linked by a shared Christian faith, decided to provide that answer. Somehow I found myself a member of that group. It was a challenge that promised adventure and offered the opportunity to help and to learn from others. It was to bring fun but also frustrations and problems, stretching people, ingenuity, limited resources and faith as we grappled with the unfamiliar, coped with extremes of climate and, initially as strangers, learned to live with each other. This is our story.

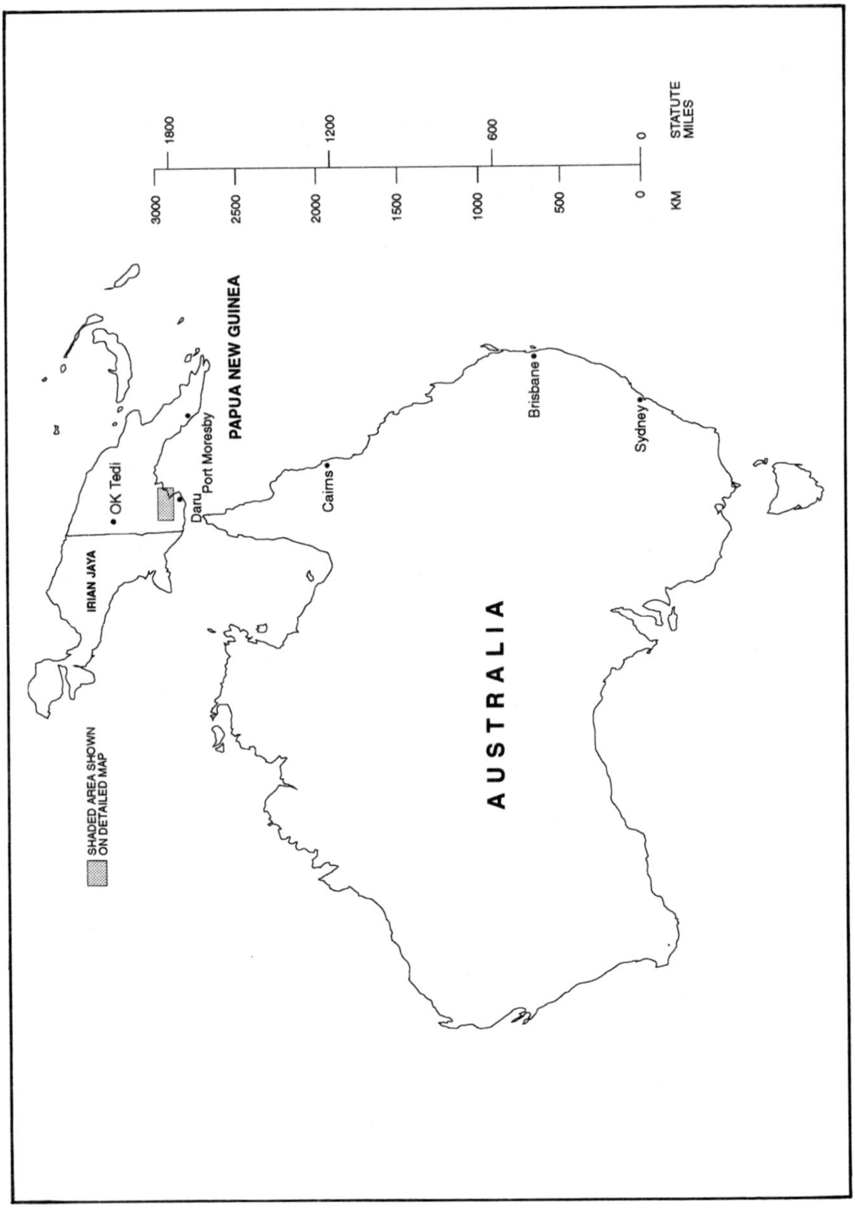
STATUTE MILES
0
600
1200
1800
KM
0
500
1000
1500
2000
2500
3000
SHADED AREA SHOWN ON DETAILED MAP
IRIAN JAYA
OK Tedi
Daru
Port Moresby
PAPUA NEW GUINEA
Cairns
Brisbane
Sydney
AUSTRALIA

1

Lift Off to Papua?

A 4 AM AWAKENING was the last thing we needed. Still jet-lagged after the journey out from the UK, we had had little sleep. Transport for our flight to Papua New Guinea was due to arrive at 5.15 am to take us to the departure point. Bleary-eyed members of the Hovercraft Expedition to PNG helped themselves to breakfast in the unfamiliar surroundings of the south block of the officers' mess at RAAF Richmond, Sydney, Australia. Others staggered around the washroom like zombies. In a helpful mood Martin Healey, who was up before four o'clock, decided to give the rest of the team a knock so they had good time to rouse themselves and get some food before leaving. The sleep-befuddled senior RAAF officer who appeared in response to the hammering on his door was not best pleased. Unknown to Martin, who thought we were the only ones there, the unfortunate chap had come in very late the previous evening.

We boarded the bus with only our flight bags; the rest of our baggage had been taken the day before, ready for loading into the Hercules C130 transport aircraft that was to take us to Papua New Guinea. Thanks to the RAAF, we were getting free transport on one of their regular training flights to PNG. Most of us had no knowledge of air force facilities and were surprised by the departure point. We had been expecting something spartan but this was like a civilian airport, carpeted with rows of seats for waiting passengers, complete with check-in, Customs and Immigration Control desks. Feeling fragile at that early hour of the morning, we slumped dozily into our seats, grateful for the quiet, orderly atmosphere.

Before long there was an announcement: 'Please make sure you do not take any prohibited items on board.' There followed a list, including 'corrosive liquids, ammunition, inflammable liquids, aerosols, pressurised gas bottles'. At that we sat up. Had not two butane cylinders been packed in a box on the pallet yesterday? 'Disposable lighters', was the next item, and that really caught our attention, to the point where consternation ensued. Several members of the team had disposable lighters intended for the anti-mosquito coils on our packing list. Now the lighters had to be surrendered. They contained pressurised liquefied gas that could explode in the low-pressure conditions of flight. A plane had crashed because of that some years before, so clearly there was a real hazard. Martin Fairley remembered having packed away one of the offending objects in a bag that already had been taken for loading into the hold of the plane. He confessed to the duty staff and was marched away to unpack his bag and remove the forbidden item. The butane gas bottles were also located and depressurised by the ground staff.

We were told the Hercules transport would be noisy, cold and uncomfortable. We would be sitting on webbing seats used by paratroopers going in for a drop, but we hoped the similarity would end there. With earplugs ready to combat the noise and warmly wrapped up, we prepared to endure the five-and-a-half-hour flight, determined to avoid using the single unisex bucket lavatory at the back of the plane, screened only by a flimsy curtain. We would be issued with a well stocked in-flight meal box as we boarded as a slight concession to comfort.

A little after 7 am we were led out to board the Hercules. The interior was a revelation. Climbing the folding metal steps on the drop-down door, we turned right into what seemed at first to be a small warehouse. The height was impressive; quilts of insulation were packed behind all the engineering hardware fixed to the walls curving above us. There was equipment everywhere.

We sat down on the rows of basic seats lining the walls and the central partition behind the crew deck. Struggling a little with the unfamiliar seatbelts, we strapped ourselves in, trying to ignore the notices about static lines for parachutes. The loadmaster, responsible for the interior of the hold, pointed out the various escape routes in case we should crash or ditch in the sea.

Almost ready for takeoff, the mere civilians among us tried to look perfectly at ease. Then as we settled back into our seats the captain emerged from the flight deck. Shaking his head in disbelief he said, 'I've just been told there is to be a twenty-four-hour delay.' We could hardly believe what we were hearing; this was worse than a scheduled airline! We had to disembark and were ushered back into the terminal to wait. Gordon Goodman, our project leader and a wing-commander in the RAF, went off to air movements control to see what information he could glean. As we waited one of the team said, 'Look at this, is someone trying to tell us something?' He was pointing at a notice that read, 'Some things were never meant to fly'.

Coming off the plane, Martin Healey had picked up a flight bag thinking someone else had left it behind, but in fact it belonged to one of the air crew and it had to be returned hurriedly before the loss was discovered. Martin had made a good start earlier. Showing considerable if suspect dexterity with an outdated plastic credit card, he had solved the problem when one of the team locked himself out of his room. For that he had been christened 'our flexible friend'. Now, with his 'bag lift' on top of the morning call gaff, it was beginning to look as though this would be one of Martin's less auspicious days.

Our waiting was interrupted by a request to report to Immigration to have our passport exit stamps cancelled. Dutifully we trooped back, not too sure whether we had left the country officially and returned or had never left at all. We were now free to return to the mess.

Later we learned the reason for our delay. Operational requirements had taken precedence over the training flight we were using. Our plane had been requisitioned for a joint operation with the Navy and would not be available until Sunday: three lost days.

There's no such thing as a free ride, they say, and the cost of ours was starting to emerge.

We had no alternative but to wait; we could not afford to pass up a free flight. The budget was tight on this privately funded expedition. For many months members of the team had been raising funds; friends, relatives and colleagues had been asked to contribute, support had been requested from churches, companies were propositioned for help in cash or kind, charitable trusts were approached for financial help. Gradually many small and moderate amounts had been accumulated to add to two significant individual contributions. Eventually the budget had just about been met, but any unforeseen expenditure would certainly tip the account into the red.

Our aim was to set up a fast hover ambulance service as a gift to the hospital at Balimo in the Western Province of Papua New Guinea (PNG). Two hovercraft were already on their way out by sea; our task at Balimo was to assemble, test and tune them, push them to the limits to prove their operational capabilities and build a base where they could be housed and maintained. National staff were to be trained to operate and maintain the hovercraft so they could operate the service after we left. Extra cost would prejudice these objectives more than delay, so we had to wait.

Some of us had already had to deal with such delays. Mike Cole, who had initiated our PNG project, had led a previous expedition taking hovercraft to the source of the Yangtze River in China. They had been held up by bureaucracy for six weeks, as Mike reminded us. His earlier expedition to Peru had been put in jeopardy for a time by the start of the Falklands War, when the British were very unpopular in South America. Setbacks were all part of the routine and something we would have to get used to.

We were an assorted bunch. Some had been together on previous expeditions and we had all met a few times at planning meetings, but most of us were strangers to each other. Yet we had volunteered to live, eat, sleep and work together for up to twelve weeks and in a demanding climate most had never experienced before. The age range of the group was wide, from late teens to early sixties, and we came from a great variety of backgrounds.

Mike Cole, a charismatic character, was our common contact. He is an inspiring enthusiast; to express even mild interest in his projects is tantamount to volunteering and signing on the dotted line. An ex-squadron leader from the RAF, Mike had for many years been involved in unusual adventures both in and out of the services. As an RAF physical education officer, he had been involved in many expeditions. During the winter of 1973, at the height of the miners' strike in England, he had been drawn into what seemed a crazy project to transport a sixteen-tonne water-drilling rig to the famine-stricken Wollo province of Ethiopia. Tear Fund, the Christian relief organisation, had provided the rig in Britain and Pat Goodland, part-time RAF chaplain and pastor of Stanmore Baptist Church, had turned to Mike for help in getting the rig to Ethiopia. With the economic problems in Britain it was hardly a good time to be looking for that sort of help, but persistence and faith prevailed and the seemingly impossible was achieved. The rig was delivered and put into service in Ethiopia, providing water for communities on the brink of extinction. Out of that experience was borne the realisation that adventure could have a purpose beyond itself, and Mike became involved in a series of humanitarian projects over a number of years.

In January 1975 Dr Bill Gould, then medical director at the Tansen Mission Hospital in West Nepal, wrote to Mike Cole. The Palpa district, where Tansen Hospital was situated, is the size of a large English county, yet it has only one road. Forming the northern boundary of the area was the Kali Gandaki River which, as Bill saw it, had the potential for health care transportation, both backwards and forwards. He said, 'Three or four days' journey could be reduced to a mere few hours.' Bill had heard about hovercraft and thought they might be suitable for turning the turbulent waters of the 'Goddess of Death', as the Nepalese called the river, into a highway of life with a 'hoverdoctor' service. He appealed to Mike for help.

So began Mike's link with hovercraft, which had led to expeditions to Nepal, Peru and China. Each expedition had a medical component, proving how suitable the craft are for delivering essential health care to isolated communities in remote parts of the world. The travelling expenses of the first two projects were covered by the Joint Services Expedition Trust, but the rest of the funds had to be raised privately. By sheer hard work, force of personality and total dependence on faith in the God he served, Mike managed to achieve wonders. Helped by men who were to become members of his teams, he gained the support of many industrial and business sponsors who contributed in cash and kind to make the expeditions possible.

The China project started almost before the expedition in Peru had finished. Dick Bell, instructor and hovercraft driver on the Peruvian expedition, records in *To the Source of the Yangtze* (Hodder & Stoughton 1991), his account of the Yangtze expedition, that even while waiting to lunch with President Belaunde at the completion of the mission in Peru, the team learned that Mike was already thinking ahead to China. Spurred on by an earlier contact with a Chinese trade delegation, he was dreaming about an expedition up previously unnavigable stretches of the Yangtze to its source. To achieve that would show that people in those remote and inhospitable areas need not be beyond the reach of medical aid. Though it would be some years coming to fruition, that dream stayed with him.

On leaving the RAF in 1986 Mike became Director of the STEP programme for the Evangelical Union of South America (EUSA, which later became Latin Link). His job was to encourage young people to give practical help to those less fortunate than themselves in South America. More than seventy projects have now been carried out, and every year a large number of young people from the UK and Australia are involved in more. The encouragement and support they give goes far beyond the work they do.

Their enthusiastic presence is in itself an enormous encouragement to those they are seeking to help, even before they lift a finger, and they certainly do more than that.

It was not until 1990, more than seven years after the Peruvian exploit, that the expedition to China became a reality. Vital major sponsorship which was being negotiated was threatened by events in Tienanmen Square in June 1989 and other problems developed, endangering the whole project. Just as things were at an impasse Mike received an invitation from Graham Zerk, an Australian doctor working in the Fly River delta of Papua New Guinea. Dr Zerk was extremely keen to have hovercraft on those rivers in order to extend the medical services there. Mike carried out a reconnaissance and found it was ideal hovercraft country. The Chinese negotiators were told that the project could be transferred to Papua New Guinea if it could not go ahead in China and they quickly concluded the deal. Once again, the foundations were in place for the next venture before preparations for the current one had been completed. Not one for dropping promising opportunities, Mike simply put the Papua possibility on one side while completing the work in China.

A magazine article on the Peru expedition, written by Bill Gould, had aroused Graham Zerk's interest when brought to his attention by his father-in-law. Bruce Olsen had also stimulated Graham's interest. Bruce, a fitter and turner by training, then ran the ECP (Evangelical Church of Papua New Guinea) mission station at Kawito on the Aramia River. He had previously experimented with hovercraft and even made a small one himself.

Working from the Balimo Hospital, Graham was acutely aware of the difficulties posed by the swamp and river systems. Time and time again, medical patrols were held up or totally frustrated in their efforts to take primary health care to the villages in the area. Vaccination and immunisation programmes had to be abandoned because making follow-up visits was impossible. Scarce time was swallowed up in battling with mud and weed on the rivers and creeks rather than caring for the sick. People's lives were put at risk or even lost because they could not get to hospital in time for effective treatment to be given. Bill Gould's article fired Graham's imagination. It seemed that the concept of a hovercraft offered many of the solutions to these problems, if not all.

Sharing these thoughts one day with Helen Brackenbury, principal of the Bible College at Mapodo on the Aramia River, Graham Zerk was amazed to learn that Helen was able to put him in touch with just the man he needed. Helen had been supported by Pat Goodland's church at Stanmore in England. The link with Pat had been kept up when he moved to a church in Herefordshire and she knew that Mike, too, was now in that area and still involved with hovercraft projects. It was a simple matter to bring together Graham Zerk's vision of an improved medical service in the Western Province of PNG and Mike's experience. That link brought about the invitation that almost diverted the Yangtze project to Papua.

Initially, everything did not go smoothly for the Papua project. There was tremendous enthusiasm from the medical staff in the field, who could see the benefits the hovercraft could bring, but some in the mission headquarters genuinely doubted whether hovercraft were the right answer. Their concern centred on the cost of purchasing the hovercraft, the imagined complexity of the vehicles and the cost of operating and maintaining them. In early 1991 these doubts led to a decision to kill off the project at birth. Those in the front line, desperately keen to reach more people more effectively, felt very frustrated by the decision.

In June 1992, Mike Cole wrote to the chairman of the ECP, which ran the hospital at Balimo, making clear that all the costs of providing two River Rover hovercraft and setting up the service would be met by the expedition. He stressed the relative simplicity of the craft and explained their modest operational cost. Reassured, the ECP gave clearance for the project in August 1992. Eighteen months' planning time would have been lost had not Mike and others continued to work on preparations for the expedition, having faith that it would go ahead. The first meeting of the expedition team took place more than two months before the final go-ahead was received from Papua.

The first I knew about the idea of an expedition to Papua New Guinea was when Mike mentioned it while showing the film of the Yangtze expedition at our church. Some time after that he asked for volunteers to join the team he was starting to form. The idea immediately appealed to me, but I considered it only for a brief time before 'reason' prevailed. It was crazy; how could I, already conscious of having too little time for all my responsibilities, have almost three months' leave from my work as a regional director of the National Trust? How would my wife, still recovering from a spinal fusion operation, manage to cope on her own? All these and other arguments quickly asserted themselves and so I quietly shelved the idea.

But some months later the project was again brought to my attention. The conviction was growing within me that this was something I should get involved in and this time the thought would not go away. Eventually I rather diffidently raised the matter with Mike Cole. Perhaps I was half hoping to be told to forget it; maybe he would suggest I was too old, as I was approaching my fifty-eighth birthday. But no, I was encouraged to give the matter some serious thought.

After a while I told my wife Kath what was running through my mind. We were both interested, yet at the same time unsure; we needed more information. At home, after church one Sunday evening, we talked things over with Mike. Unwisely I expressed some mild interest when Mike mentioned that he wanted someone to write a book on the expedition. I ought to have known better. By the time I went to Mike's home a week later to meet other possible members of the team, I was committed to the project – in it up to my neck, despite the fact that I still had to ask my employers if I could be released.

The room was full when I arrived. As I sank into the one remaining chair I glanced around at those who would be my companions. They were a varied bunch with a wide age range from early twenties to late middle age. For most of the idea was still a dream to be worked out, but there was enormous enthusiasm.

Rarely have I attended a meeting with such a quietly positive approach to a task. We knew it would not be easy; the potential problems and hazards involved were too great. But we could call upon experienced professionals who had taken part in earlier expeditions. And we had our shared Christian faith.

As I listened to Mike, I became aware of the wealth of experience built up by members of the earlier expeditions. Mike himself had the main fund of knowledge, but he was well supported by Steve Moody, whose wide engineering experience of the hovercraft would be invaluable, as well as by the doctors, Ray (Rachel) Pinniger and Bill Gould, both of whom had extensive experience in medical missionary work, Ray in Bhutan and Bill in Nepal.

Listening to the health briefing by Bill Gould could have been worrying had it not been obvious that this was not just textbook knowledge but was also drawn from solid, direct and practical experience. The thought that we should have such a high level of experience and knowledge available to us was very comforting as we heard – most of us for the first time – of the health hazards we would be facing. Poisonous snakes, cholera, hepatitis, malaria were but a few.

Over lunch we began to get to know our potential partners on the expedition, as well as to reflect that the catering in PNG would be unlikely to be as good as that provided by Mike's wife Jackie. The stunning views out from High Rising, west towards the Black Mountains or north-east to the Malverns, would also give way to something entirely different in Papua which most of us could visualise only from the slides we had seen that morning. Some of the pictures had been taken by Jeff Goulding, a young farmer from nearby Gorsley Baptist Church, who had gone out in October 1991 with Ray Pinniger to make a preliminary assessment of the project. He would not be coming to PNG, but would be our liaison man at Gorsley.

Tasks were tentatively allocated during the course of the day. Those of the doctors and the two women, Aileen Boyd and Sarah Williams, both medical students, were obvious. Michael Pinkess was identified as our potential purse holder. He had recently retired from Bowring Aviation, our sponsors and expedition insurers, and his experience as an insurance broker would be useful. Administration and planning, assisting both at home and on location, was assigned to Gordon Goodman (then head of the RAF Navigation School), who would take over from Mike as field operations leader in Papua New Guinea. This would release Mike to pay a visit to South America to oversee some aspects of the STEP teams. Radio links would be of vital importance to our task, so it was good to know we had an electronics expert in the person of Jonathan Allan, a young research engineer. (Later, Martin Fairley, another electronic systems man, took over that role, so releasing Jonathan for video work, which was also in his line.) In view of his earlier experience, the bulk of the engineering work automatically went to Steve Moody. I, of course, was given the task of scribe; my early training and experience as a building surveyor would also be of use. So the first structure began to emerge, giving us all an idea of the role we were to play and our responsibilities to one another.

Everyone had to find a way to make the time needed for the expedition. Some gave up work in order to be available; others scraped together a combination of holiday time and unpaid leave. Jonathan Allan took advantage of a voluntary redundancy scheme and hoped to find suitable work on returning; Steve Moody committed himself to joining the project as soon as possible after the birth of the baby his wife was expecting in March. Sarah Williams and Aileen Boyd took the opportunity to combine the expedition with the 'elective' element of their final year medical training, while Gordon Goodman managed to get seven months' leave of absence from the RAF so he would be free to deal with initial planning, as well as leading in the field during Mike Cole's absence in South America.

It would be a little while yet before Mike knew the precise composition of his team, but he was already deeply involved in negotiations and planning the early stages of the project. During the first team meeting there had been some encouragement. Laurie Humphrey and Andrew Schache had called from Queensland as the meeting began to say that they were fully committed to the project. We needed them to play a key part in the building work and their timely call was a great endorsement of our faith. It was faith that was taking Mike forward, strong in the conviction that God had a task ready for us, and that all we had to do was be willing to play our part. He had taken that as a theme in his opening remarks to the group, basing his comments on a verse in the letter written by the Apostle Paul to the church at Ephesus: 'For we are God's workmanship, created in Christ Jesus to do good works, which God prepared in advance for us to do' (Ephesians 2:10 NIV).

Faith and works must go together. We definitely needed practical support and already Mike had been working hard. He sent a note to all the potential PNG team members bringing us up to date with progress before he flew out to South America for six weeks to oversee the operations of the ten STEP teams working there. Mike was negotiating with several airlines over concessionary travel rates for the team to and from Australia. The Bank Line was likely to provide free shipping for the two hovercraft, and Clark's, the footwear manufacturers, had offered to provide the whole team with stout shoes, very necessary to guard against the possibility of snakebite. The first River Rover was already paid for, thanks to a generous gift. Still, that was only a start; there was a way to go yet and individual team members were expected to play their part in raising sponsorship and donations.

Many of us were becoming aware of aspects of the project that would be very different from our everyday life. I am something of a loner, used to a position of leadership: how would I fit in as a team member? Accustomed, possibly even needing, to spend some time each day alone, how would I deal with being with others virtually all day, every day? Each member of the team had his or her own particular circumstances to face.

It would be easy, or at least convenient, to pretend these issues did not exist. These were the points at which our own natural self-interest came face to face with an opportunity for practical service. To go for no other reason than simply wanting to have an 'adventure' would deny that opportunity, even if, to the casual observer, what we were offering seemed to be the same. For us, unless we went in the spirit of Christ, it would be hypocritical.

A scene from a Billy Graham film I had seen many years before came to mind. Driving across the airfield towards a small aeroplane, Dr Graham was stopped and challenged by a security guard, who demanded: 'Where do you think *you're* going, for Christ's sake?' Through the open car window Billy Graham smiled and replied, 'Friend, I go everywhere for Christ's sake.' His seemed a good example to follow.

Toward the end of August, the whole team was confronted with more realities of being involved. Like a needle from the blue came a letter from Bill Gould and Ray Pinniger, our medics on the team, setting out the health precautions that had to be started immediately, even though our departure was still six months away. For most of the team it meant two or three injections every month up to departure, and a routine of anti-malarial treatment that would start before we left and continue during the expedition and for six weeks after our return. This was, we felt, a small price to pay if it protected us against serious illness while we were away. It was also a salutary reminder of the difference in the health care we had to hand compared to that available to the Gogodala people we were going to help.

A serious health concern arose while Mike was away in South America looking after the STEP programme; his wife Jackie was diagnosed as suffering from multiple sclerosis. Treatment improved her condition but still left her rather unwell. The implications for the future were potentially serious for both Jackie and Mike. We should have to bear them up in prayer.

Mike returned to the UK a little earlier so he and Jackie could spend a few days together before he launched into a busy weekend programme of meetings in Tonbridge in mid-September. These had been arranged jointly by Tonbridge Baptist Church and the Anglican churches of the Tonbridge parish. Four meetings in two days told young people, their parents and others about the work and challenge of the STEP programme and also launched the planned expedition to Papua New Guinea.

The Tonbridge weekend started off with a breakfast meeting attended by about seventy men from various churches in the area. Fortified by breakfast, they listened for over an hour to Mike's gripping accounts of the STEP projects and earlier expeditions. Typically, Mike was bubbling over with anecdotes about the difficulties faced and overcome, often by the most unconventional means; linking modern technology and the needs of undeveloped areas is not always easy, but it can be done. Nothing illustrated this better than the story Mike told of the problem of transporting vital vaccines to remote parts of Tibet. Vaccines have to be kept at specific temperatures in transit and storage to retain their potency, and refrigeration is essential. Without it the remote areas of Tibet had no vaccination programme.

To overcome the problem, solar power was linked to small refrigerators. A vet who was a member of the expedition team advised on modifications to the traditional panniers used for carrying loads on the yak, the beast of all burden in Tibet. A refrigerator was fixed on one side of the pannier, batteries on the other and a solar panel on top. Mounted on a yak, this Heath Robinson blend of modern and traditional methods worked well, providing a means of carrying vaccines in good condition into the most farflung areas. We realised we might well require similar ingenuity in PNG.

The meeting generated much enthusiasm and produced a recruit for PNG in the person of Brian Black. He had given up his former garage and car sales business and decided to join the team. For me, the quote of the weekend was Mike talking about moving his audio-visual equipment to his next speaking location. 'We'll do it in slow time,' he said. As Mike always seems to do everything at the double, 'slow time' was an impossible concept to link with him.

While our attention centred on the delta area where we were to operate, it was fascinating to learn about the wonderful island of which it was but a part. It is little more than 120 years since Europeans actually settled in New Guinea. Just over sixty years ago, more than one million people were discovered living in the Eastern Highlands of Papua. They were totally unaware of the rest of the world, unaware even of what lay beyond the mountains forming the horizon of their high-plateau universe.

The exposure of the highlanders to the advances of what we in a superior way call 'civilisation' has been dramatic in the extreme. Tales are still told of first contact with the 'white men', whom they believed to be spirits returning from the dead, with the *bois* (black coastal New Guineans acting as bearers) thought to be dead relatives of the highlanders in spirit form. Goroka, the capital of the Eastern Highlands Province, which in 1930 did not exist, was a flourishing town by 1980. According to Bob Connolly and Robyn Anderson, the Australian film makers whose documentary *First Contact* brought knowledge of this area to a wider audience, it had 'schools, a university, a teachers' college, police barracks and courthouses, tourist hotels, cinema, supermarkets, beer garden, coffee-processing plant, churches, airport, bowling green and cricket pitch, highlander coffee barons, labourers and lawyers, streets lined with Japanese four-wheel drive vehicles and a hospital treating highlanders for such diverse ills as heart disease and arrow wounds'.

Papua New Guinea is an area still largely undocumented. So much more is waiting to be discovered. For its size the island has more mountains, swamps and jungle than any comparable region on earth. The 12,000 or so recorded species of flowering plants are thought to be less than two-thirds of the potential total number present on the island. The four main river systems of the island pour vast quantities of water and silt into the sea every day. In *New Guinea*, his study of the island, Roy D. Mackay has estimated that the Fly River alone pours enough water into the sea each day to provide ten gallons (forty-five litres) of water for each person on earth. Vast areas of the country are still mapped only in outline, with much detail yet to be filled in. So much about Papua New Guinea seems larger than life, with at least 250 species of rhododendron and more than 2500 species of orchids including the giant strap-leafed *Vandopsis* with its three-foot (one-metre) long leaves and ten-foot (three-metre) long spray of blooms. More than 1000 species of fish have been listed off its shores, with possibly as many again yet to be discovered. Its skies are populated by 700 species of bird, a similar number to Australia which is ten times larger. Notable among its insect species is the largest moth in the world, the Hercules moth, with its forty square inch (two hundred and fifty square centimetre) wing area, and here again only one-

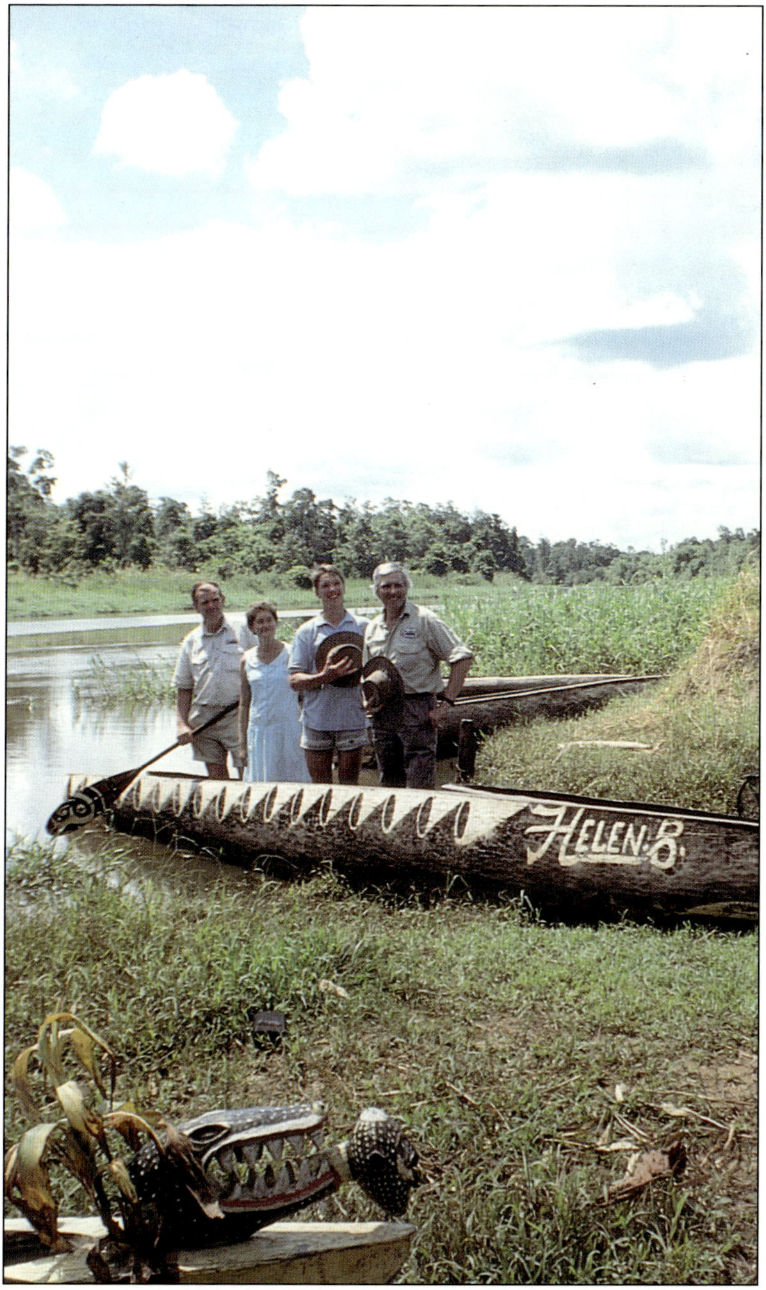

Birth of the expedition - Gorsley men with
the Helen Brackenbury canoe.

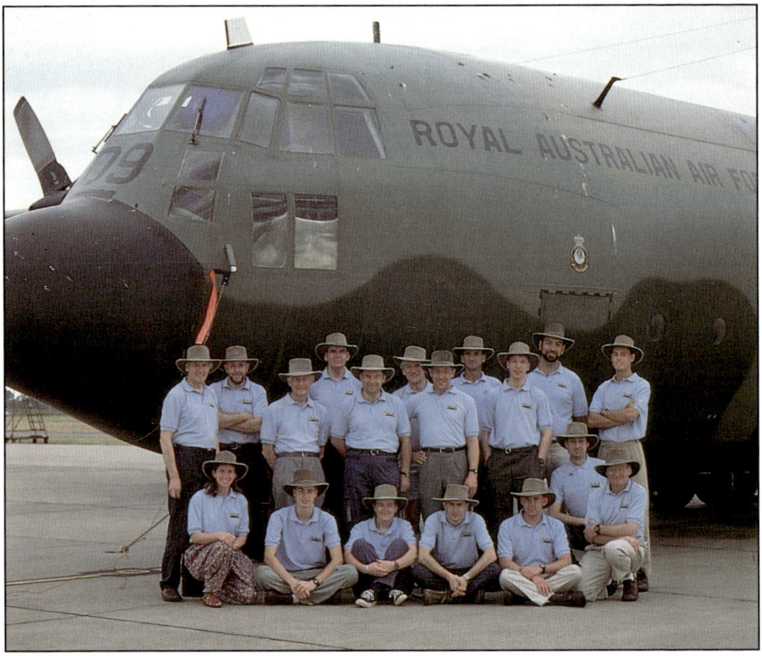

Above: RAAF Hercules *Below:* Dawn liftoff with MAF

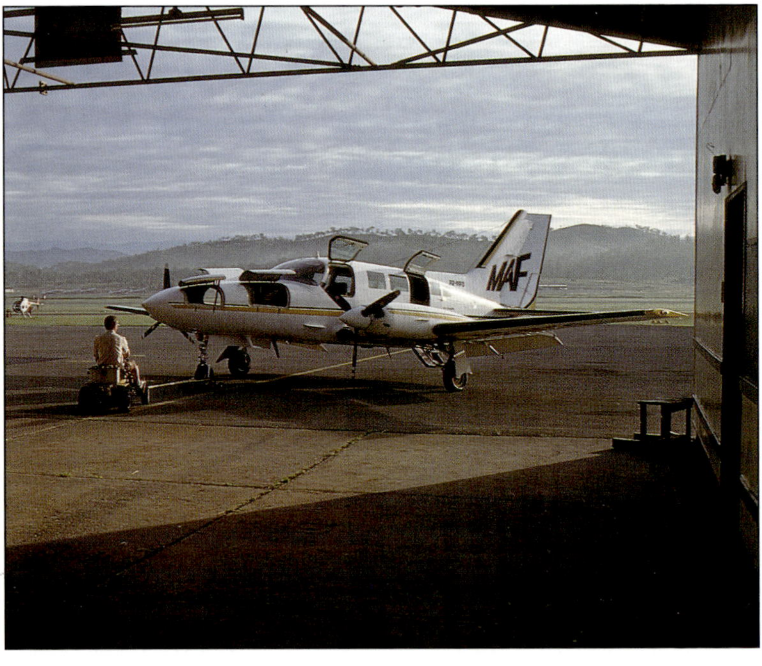

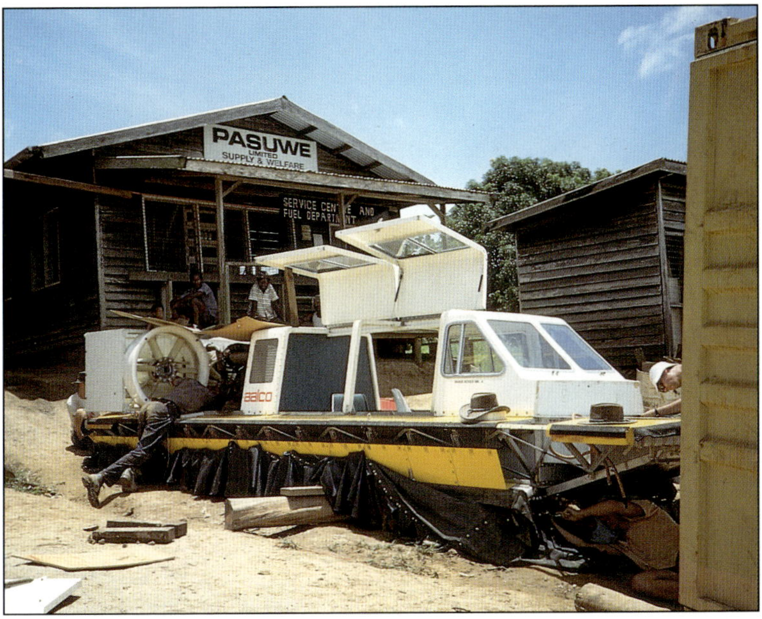

Above: Putting it all together at Kawaito in 113°F (45°C) heat
Below: Launch of River Rover 401, *Dr Andrew Baur*
Overpage: The grass-clogged Balimo lagoon

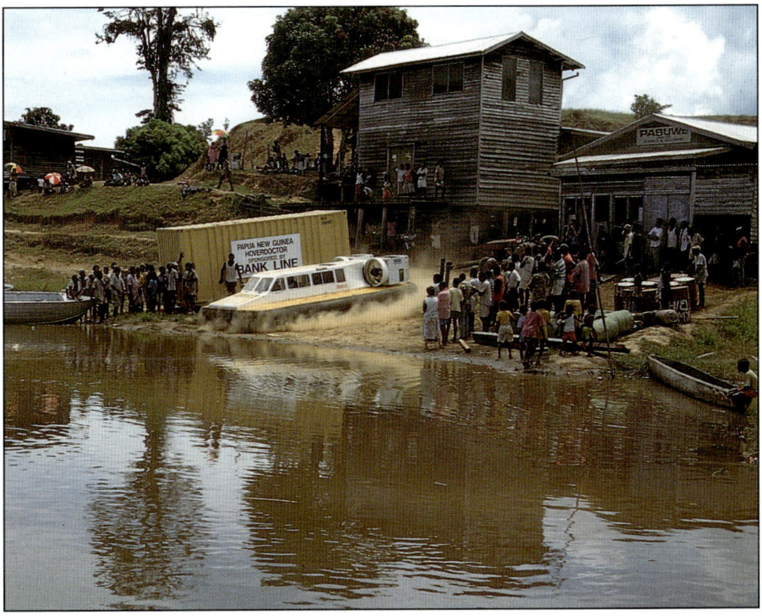

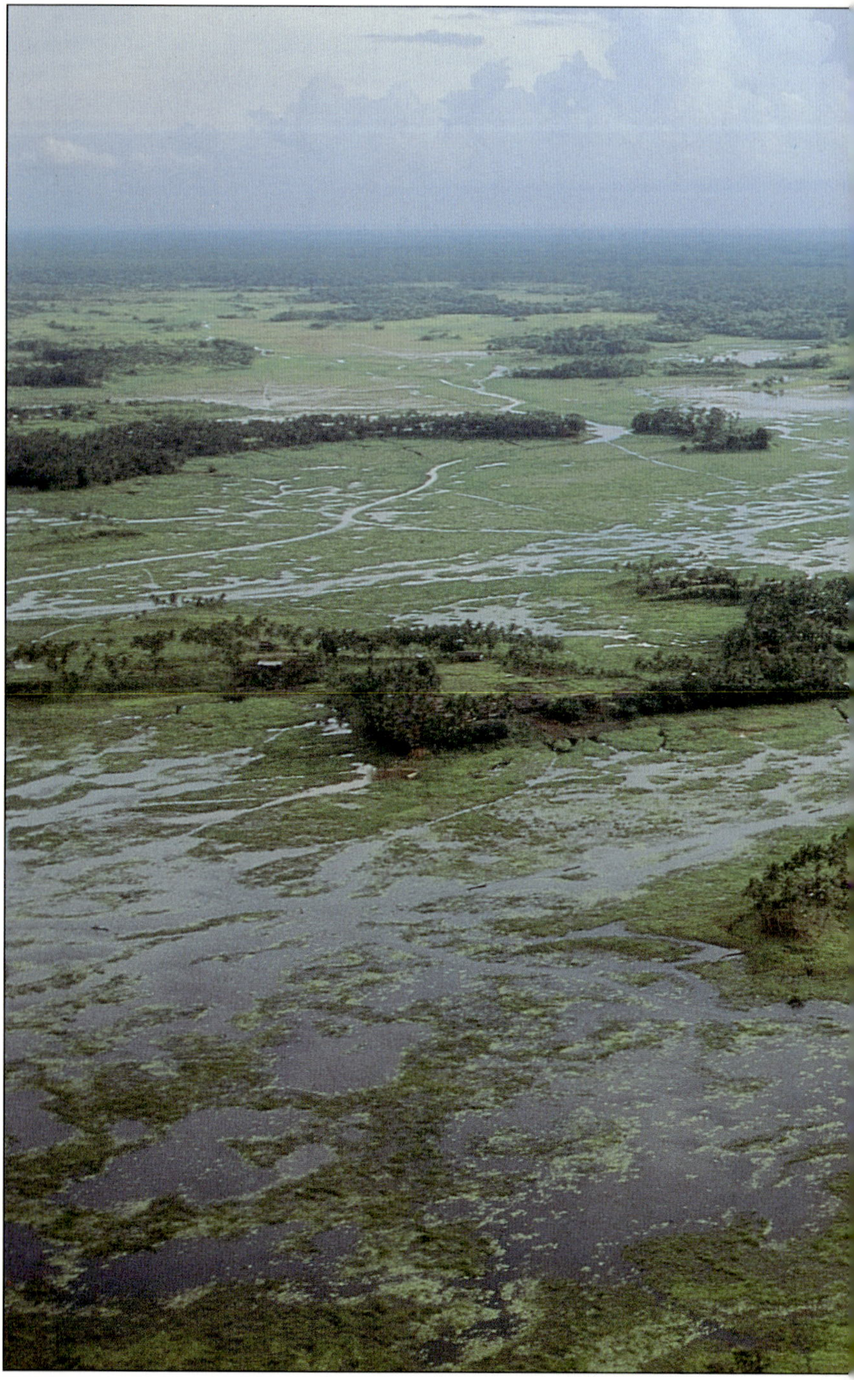

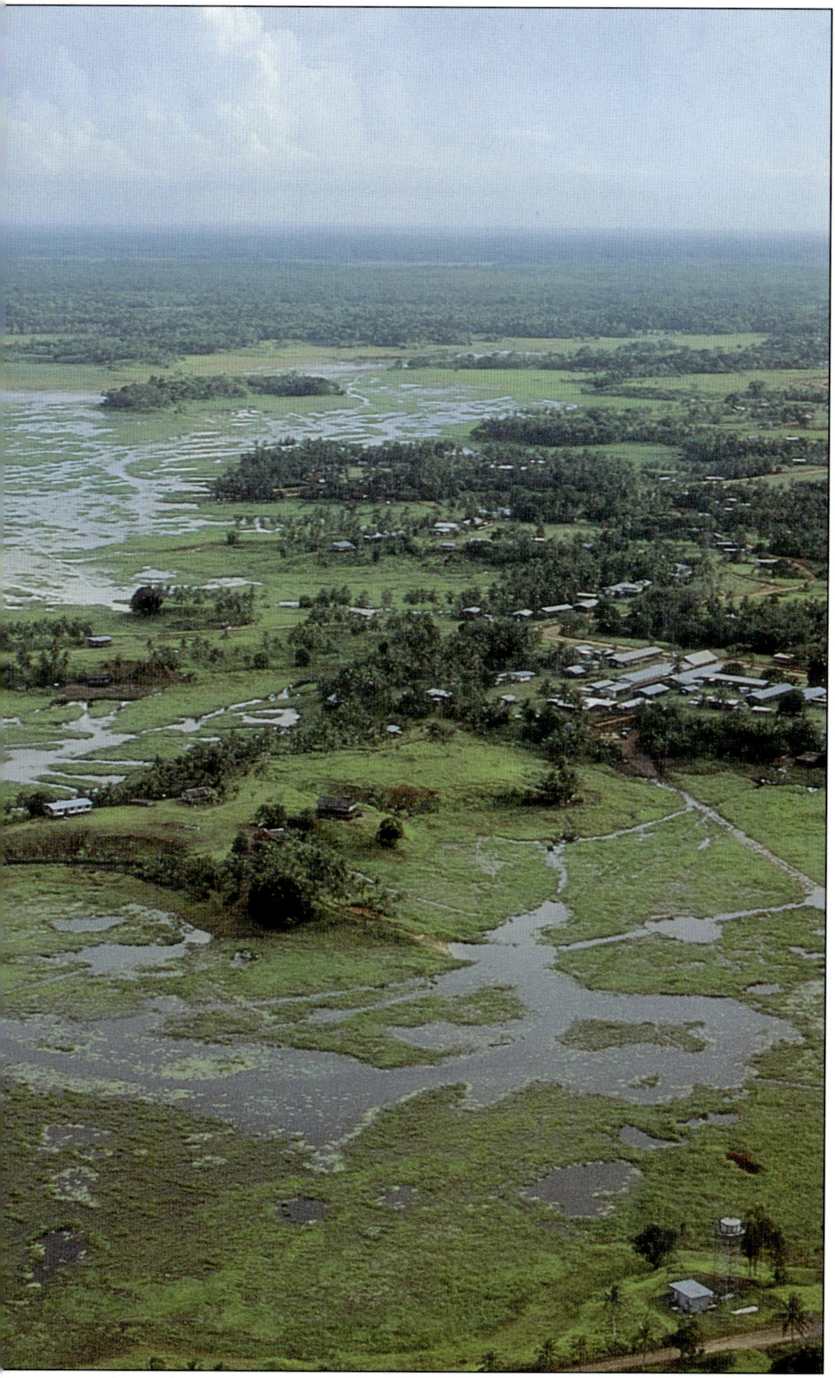

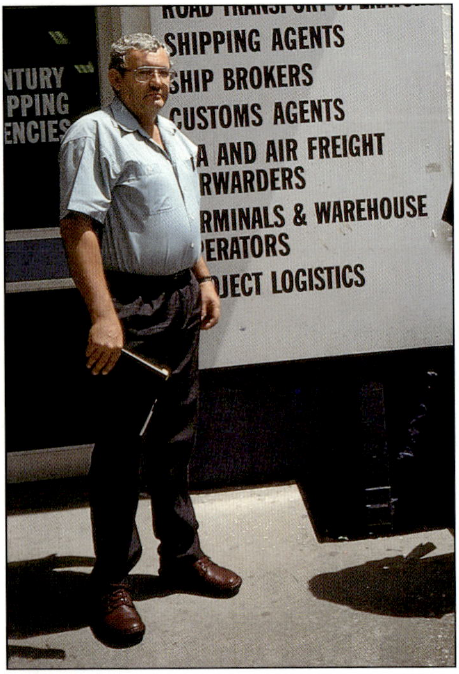

Left: Bruce Olsen, our man in Port Moresby
Below: 401 arrives at Balimo to a tumultuous welcome
Right: Pre-launch testing of 402 at Port Moresby
Below right: Off loading the easy way at Coconut Island, Balimo

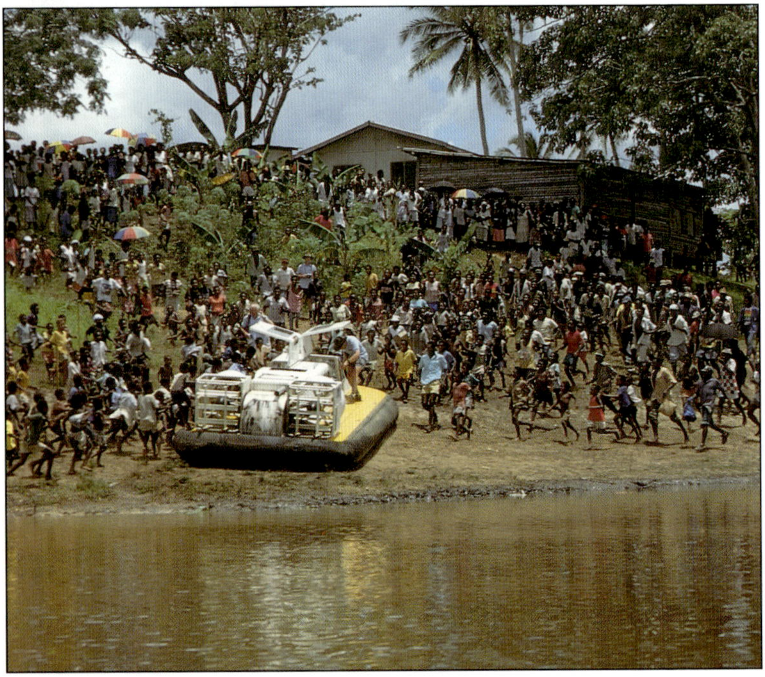

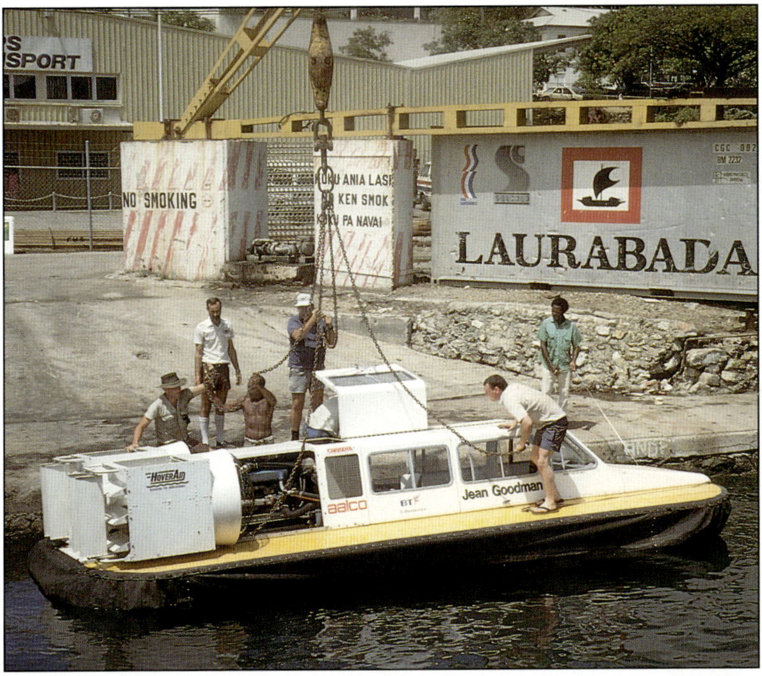
NO SMOKING
LAURABADA
HoverAid
aalco
BT
Jean Goodman

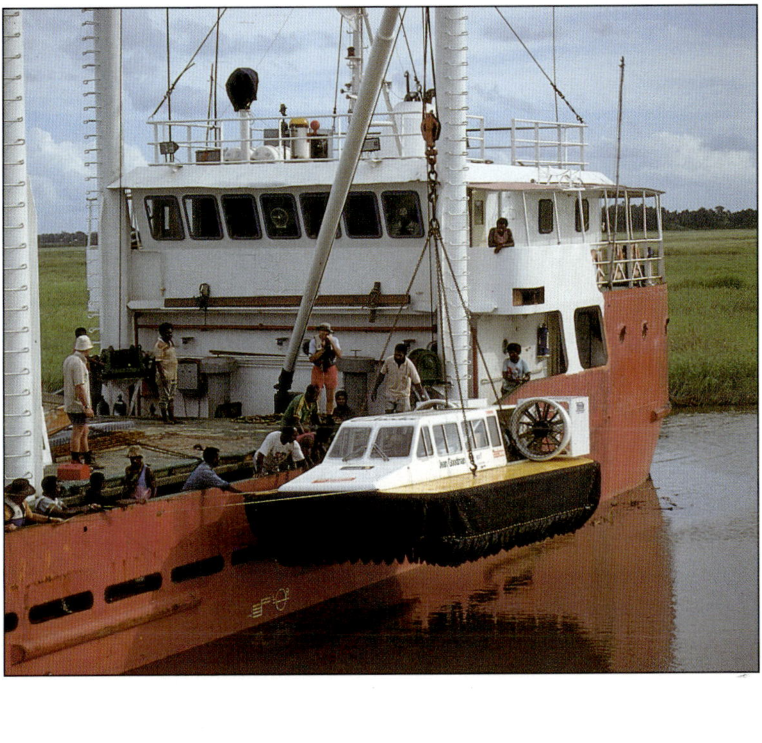

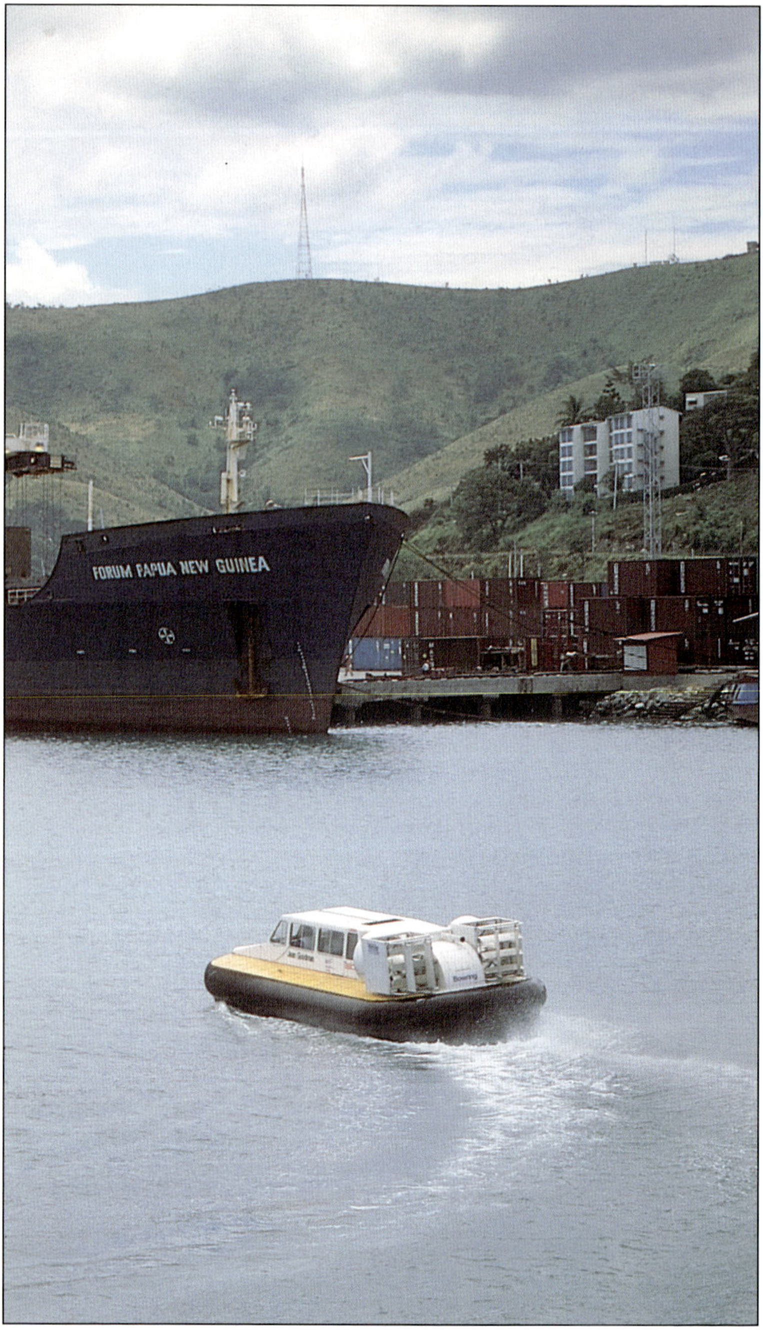

Media and VIP demonstration, Port Moresby harbour

third of the insect species are thought to have been listed so far.

The mountains are the major physical feature of New Guinea, containing the highest peaks of the Orient outside the Himalayas. In Irian Jaya, the Indonesian western part of the island of New Guinea, there are snow-topped mountains only 400 miles (640 kilometres) or so south of the equator, the highest, Carstenz Toppen, rising to 16,500 feet (5029 metres). It is run a close second in Papua New Guinea by Mount Wilhelm at 15,400 feet (4694 metres). In the trans-Fly area the peaks do not dominate and there is no word for 'mountain' in the language of the local tribes. However, even there, the effect of the mountain ranges on the climate is significant. Monsoons and trade winds forced up the mountains condense out their moisture as rain that forms the rushing torrents carrying thousands of tonnes of silt down to the coastal plains and swamps, and up to forty miles (about sixty kilometres) out to the sea. Yet Roy D. Mackay records walking in areas of heavy forest in the Southern Highlands and Western Province where everything underfoot is bone dry, despite the appearance of the lush vegetation. The limestone plateau on which the vegetation thrives is so porous that it soaks up the heavy rain falling on it.

These are some of the wonders of creation we were to experience in Papua New Guinea, features that could only serve to emphasise the awesome nature of the Creator God we wanted to serve. The prospect was a thrilling one and brought us a sense of privilege. No wonder we were looking forward to our departure.

2

Destination Balimo

SNOW WAS FALLING as we arrived at Heathrow airport early in the evening of 27 February 1993. The group assembled as one by one members arrived from various parts of the country. Our plans and preparations had been building up to this moment and there was an air of excitement as we greeted each other. Only twelve were flying out at this time; others would join us en route to PNG. Gordon Goodman and Brian Black had gone ahead as an advance party and Jonathan Allan was already in Australia on a pre-expedition holiday. He would meet us in Sydney along with Graeme Bencke and Jenny Smith. Graeme, a young flying officer in the RAF awaiting pilot training, had been on leave in Australia when, like Gordon, he had been given leave of absence to take part in the expedition. Immediately, Gordon used him as our man on the spot to help prepare the way for us. Jenny, born in Australia and brought up there and in PNG, had gone ahead for a brief visit to her family leaving Gareth, her husband and also a member of the team, to follow. Jenny had a varied background with many skills, including rounding up sheep on a motorcycle as a jillaroo on one of the massive outback sheep stations.

The mound of baggage was growing, some being redistributed as different members arrived. Gareth was busy passing round the five hundred cost-price Fujichrome films he had obtained. John Field, a transportation engineer, distributed a quantity of water purifiers and Michael Pinkess handed out umbrellas and sun hats from Legal & General, one of our sponsors. An unwieldy ten-foot (three-metre) whip aerial was added to the pile by Mike Cole who had picked up various items of radio equipment on the way to the airport.

'Stuff this in your bag,' said Mike, putting a box into my hand.

'But where?' I protested, looking at a bursting rucksack.

'Well, we've got to get them in somewhere,' was his reply as he went off to unload more of his electronic paraphernalia.

As soon as the whole group had assembled, we moved over to the security check area. The only items that excited interest were the assorted penknives the group carried as part of the expedition gear; these had to be handed over for scrutiny. Check-in was next. Singapore Airlines had agreed to sponsor the expedition by giving us a special party-rate discount. Looking at the thirty-seven pieces of baggage the twelve of us had amassed, I hoped their staff were not about to regret their generosity. They coped splendidly and soon had the lot consigned to a single container to await us at Sydney, so we did not have to go through the whole business again at our Singapore stopover.

We had some time in hand before we boarded. Relatives were having a last cup of tea with members of the team before saying goodbye and other farewells were being said by telephone. For the moment the sense of excitement and adventure was overlaid by the parting. Mike, seasoned by many previous experiences, was already carrying out his job by having a last-minute conference with Chris Powell and his team. They were negotiating to make a TV film of the expedition and were hoping to join us in PNG.

Boarding formalities over, we were soon airborne and Kath and I settled into our seats. She was travelling with me as far as Singapore on her way to Australia. In front of us were Tim Goulding and Ben Oliver. At nineteen years of age they were the youngest members of the party and were clearly enjoying the luxury of the attention carefully lavished upon us by the Singapore Airlines cabin staff. Tim, a young farmer from Herefordshire was, like Mike Cole and me, a member of Gorsley Baptist Church. For him this journey was a novel experience. Jeff, his cousin, had once jokingly described him as 'never having been east of Cheltenham'. Ben was a budding engineer having a year out before going to Cambridge. He had been gaining practical experience by helping to build our two River Rover hovercraft and was about to put that experience to good use.

Only a few hours into the flight, Tim started to feel unwell. Having our own doctor travelling with us was handy for, diagnosing a rapid allergic reaction, Bill Gould treated Tim accordingly and within a few hours his condition improved.

Stepping from the air-conditioned airport terminal into the dark humid Singapore night was like walking into a warm wet sponge, a total contrast to the cold, snowy London evening we had left behind. Thrown by the time change, most of us had little sleep. After breakfast we gathered for a brief time of devotion led by Mike. This was our first morning together so we wanted to set our pattern for the future. Then, with time to spare before our evening flight, we were glad to spend a few hours wandering around the older parts of the city in the Indian and Chinese areas.

By evening we were more than ready to be on our way. At the

airport Kath and I were to part; she was flying to Melbourne and I, with the team, was bound for Sydney. Our departure gates lay in opposite directions. We said goodbye quickly, turned our backs on each other and went our separate ways. Our farewell was harder than I had envisaged as I rejoined the team.

With only hand luggage, formalities were few and we were soon on the second stage of our journey. Despite the care of the airline staff at Heathrow, we were lacking one of our bags when we arrived at Sydney. Unfortunately it was young Tim's rucksack. Being new to international travel and unwell on the first part of the journey, Tim understandably felt that having luggage go astray was not a good start to his adventure.

Emerging into the Sydney sunshine we were met by Gordon Goodman and Graeme Bencke. Richmond RAAF base was our next destination but with only two hired cars for transport, the new arrivals and some of the baggage had to travel by train with the rest of the bags going by car. Martin Fairley and I volunteered to take the luggage by train, leaving most of the team to go sightseeing in Sydney and travel out later.

Dumped in the booking hall of a suburban station with countless heavy bags and packages, Martin and I looked at each other helplessly. We had taken on a mammoth task. With a great effort we got on the train complete with baggage, helped by the platform hand and a young Australian woman named Tilly. Seeing our struggles she got off the train to help us and, finding that we had not a clue when we should arrive at our station, she insisted on travelling beyond her own stop to ensure that we got off at the right place.

In the surprising way that complete strangers can, when travelling, Tilly told us her story. Left to look after her divorced alcoholic father, she was at heart a lonely girl feeling totally rejected by her mother. Reaching our station Tilly helped us off with our load and continued chatting until her return train arrived. Thanking her as we said goodbye I slipped a Gideon New Testament into her hand, telling her of the helpful references in the early pages. We should not be around to befriend her any more but in a paraphrase of the UK advertisement 'we knew a man who could', and the Testament introduced Him.

Richmond air base is huge. We were driven deep into the heart of it to the officers' mess where we were staying and soon the rest of the team arrived from their sightseeing trip and started to settle in. Laurie Humphrey and Andrew Schache had also arrived. Queenslanders and good friends used to working together, they had both worked on the mission station at Balimo for a time. Laurie, a carpenter and builder, had designed the building we were to construct at Balimo. Andrew, a genial giant of a man, could turn his hand to almost any practical task. Helped by my building surveying background, I quickly formed an affinity with them. In no time we were on to building matters and found we spoke the same language, even if with distinctly different accents.

Next we civilians had to be inducted into some of the mess etiquette. Dress in the dining room had to conform to certain standards. We were also instructed that on first entering the reception area we were to sign in, using the book there for that purpose. I signed in beneath the signature of an air vice-marshal, Mike Cole following my example. It was only later we discovered that we had used the distinguished visitors' book, and not the record book! I wonder what the next air vice-marshal made of signing below a mere Mr and a lowly squadron-leader?

We were due to leave in the Hercules transport at an early hour the following morning – or so we thought – giving no time for photo sessions beforehand. So, the day before, with time to spare, we trooped off for team photos in front of one of the large planes. We had to be escorted while on the operational area of the base and on our arrival at 36 Squadron's headquarters, Flight-Lieutenant Linda Corbould took us in hand. She had been in the RAAF for twelve years, having joined air traffic control straight from school, and was now a Hercules pilot. Tall, slim, dressed in a flying suit with her auburn hair in a single simple plait at the back, her lively personality quickly became evident as she led us across the airfield to the planes. The badge she wore with her pilot's wings carried the description 'Girl'; it hardly seemed necessary. Graeme Benke produced *Crocodile Dundee* style 'genuine steerhide' hats for each member of the team and we posed for a photograph for the sponsor who had supplied them. Linda expertly handled about half a dozen cameras thrust on her by different members of the team, firing them off in rapid succession. Back at the Squadron HQ we also collected some up-to-date full-colour maps of the area where we should be operating. In anticipation of our departure next morning we went off in good spirits for our evening meal.

One of the mess rules was that diners filled up spaces at the tables in turn as they arrived, so that one found oneself seated next tocomplete strangers. At our table that evening was a group from the Australian Army Rifle Association. The young woman on my left, belying her civilian dress, was a lieutenant and a member of the rifle team due to be competing in England during July at Bisley, Gloucestershire, not far from my home.

While we were travelling out to Australia, Brian Black was already at work in Port Moresby, the capital of Papua New Guinea, having flown directly there as a one-man advance party. Gordon had thought him well suited to making local arrangements in Moresby, knowing of his business experience as a former garage owner. He was also given the task of overseeing the arrival of the container in which the first of our two hovercraft had been shipped. Packed with the hovercraft was a large quantity of tinned and dried food, tools and other items that we should need as soon as we arrived at Balimo. The container had been shipped out to Port Moresby from the UK by the Bank Line, one of our sponsors. It was to be transferred to a smaller vessel, the *Agutoi Chief*, for the journey across the Gulf of Papua and up the Bamu and Aramia rivers to Kawito. Although only six miles (ten kilometres) or so apart, the distance from Kawito to Balimo by water was more than half as far again due to the twists and bends of the river and lagoon channels. The supplies had to be taken by barge on that final stage as boats of the size of the *Agutoi Chief* could not get into the lagoon at Balimo. That involved many trips, as the barge could only carry ten tonnes at a time.

Life had been hectic from the moment Brian arrived. He had been met by Bruce Olsen, one of the ECP missionaries in Port Moresby. After thirty-two hours of travel, Brian was whisked almost directly off the plane to a press conference about the expedition. At least, that had been the intention; he had found himself totally upstaged by the sudden outbreak of hostilities on Bougainville Island off the east coast of PNG and the press conference had been postponed. The British High Commissioner's office had to be contacted, as did the local representatives of a number of our sponsors. Building supplies had to be ordered and loaded onto the *Agutoi Chief*, bread and fresh fruit had to be sent in advance to Balimo. Barbara Fergusson, our staunch supporter from Salisbury, had arrived by then and went on with the supplies by plane, leaving Brian to follow the next day.

Next came the fun of trying to offload the heavy steel container at Kawito. It was far from easy with no dockside facilities to aid the transfer from ship to river bank. Eventually, the container and fifty-three drums of gravel were on shore. The sundry supplies were to be transported to Balimo and the hovercraft was to await assembly so it could then be launched and driven under its own power.

After the debacle of our retreat from the Hercules and the subsequent delay at Richmond, we had time on our hands and no plans to fill it. That state of affairs was not allowed to exist for long; Dick Bell was roped in to give us a lecture on the theoretical aspects of driving the hovercraft. He had not expected to do that until we were in PNG. A former RAF Lightning test pilot and a veteran of the Yangtze expedition when he had been chief hovercraft pilot, Dick Bell was better qualified than anyone to do that.

Listening to Dick is never boring. A colourful character, bubbling over with faith, fervour and fun, he is one of the most extroverted people I have ever met. With him, everything is larger than life. One day he was making some tea and offered Laurie a cup.

'How do you like your tea, Laurie?' he asked.

'Oh, just medium, Dick.'

There was a long pause. 'I don't think I can handle medium,' said Dick, thoughtfully.

'You've said it, Bell. You can't handle medium, that really sums you up!' said Mike, Dick's close friend for many years.

Dick took all this with his typical cheery grin.

The next day we profited from the delay by making a trip into Sydney. While the city itself attracted some, others were all for making the most of the sunshine by heading for the beach. Arrangements were made to hire a minibus for the next day to take us west of the city to the Blue Mountains for a trip to the Jenolan limestone caves.

In the meantime, one serious omission in our equipment had come to light. We did not have a large teapot! Consequently four of us were given the vital mission of acquiring a suitable one on the way to the mountains, in Rachel Grimmer's car. Rachel had joined the expedition as an RAAF nominee. A doctor in the RAAF she was to prove a most welcome addition to our team. Married to a Hercules pilot, she was based at Richmond and so knew all the routines at the base, which was of great advantage to us.

We enjoyed the scenery of the Blue Mountains and the cool atmosphere of the caves as a welcome respite from the hot sun outside. It seemed strange being tourists for the day when we had expected to be in PNG on our way to Balimo. At the billet on our return there was a welcome message for us from Singapore Airlines that Tim's rucksack had been located. It had been wrongly labelled and was awaiting a Mr Spalding in Sydney.

We anticipated a 4 am start the following morning and arrived early at the departure point for what we hoped would be a successful leave-taking of Richmond air base, much though we had appreciated its hospitality. Shortly after seven o'clock we were airborne.

By one o'clock that afternoon we had reached Papua New Guinea at last and were looking around for all the usual entry procedures. There were none; not a single official appeared. After a long delay Bruce Olsen, who had arrived to meet us, went off to check and returned to say, 'There's no one from Customs or Immigration here. They're all over on the civilian side dealing with a large planeload of passengers.'

We really appreciated the wonderful friendly welcome we received from Bruce and from Ron Smith. In no time at all we arrived at the mission houses at Waigani. There we had another warm welcome from Kharen, Bruce's wife, and from Bernard and Linda Lewis, their neighbours and fellow missionaries. Quickly, we were distributed among their two houses and a third that was kept for missionaries and others like ourselves in transit. Tea, cold drinks and cake drew us out into the garden and soon we were tucking into the food they had prepared for us.

Later Ron slipped away and shortly reappeared with an impressive electronic keyboard on which he then gave a wonderful performance of hymn tunes and spiritual songs. Soon, and easily, we moved into a time of fellowship together, giving thanks for all that our Lord had done for us. Bruce had a barbecue going, darkness was falling, lights were switched on in the trees overhead and we enjoyed the food and the relaxed friendly atmosphere. It was a good first experience of Papua New Guinea.

The next morning, we were Balimo bound at last; at least, six of us were. Because of the delays, we should have to fly out in relays, in a smaller plane than originally planned. Mission Aviation Fellowship (MAF) were splendid in rescheduling for us. Andrew, Laurie, Gordon, Gareth and Jenny and I formed the first party. Gordon was delighted to have the co-pilot's seat. The MAF Islander was rather different from the RAF Phantoms he had been used to, but he was clearly pleased to be at the business end again.

We took off shortly after eight for a two-and-a-quarter-hour flight out across the Gulf of Papua, over the mouth of the Bamu

River, in sight of the mighty Fly River and across the low-lying land of the Fly delta area to the lagoons of Balimo. Every day the Fly is said to pour into the sea ten gallons (forty-five litres) of water for everyone living on the earth, but the turbulent power of those mighty forces were masked by the quiescent landscape below, as we flew into Balimo looking in vain for the huge, open-water lagoon areas we were expecting to see. The only water visible was in narrow channels winding tortuously through large areas of mid-green, bounded by seemingly endless jungle. These, we found, were the lagoons. Sometimes like large inland seas, they were showing a different face this year, the grass triumphant, blocking off the open water and forcing the canoe users to follow an intricate maze of water channels. This was the real barrier to rapid progress that the hovercraft had to defeat if they were to provide the lifesaving service we had come to give.

Dropping down through the low-lying broken cloud, the pilot flew over the airstrip and made a visual check that it was clear before turning to run in for the landing. There were no hi-tech aids on this grass airfield. The arrivals area was no more than a simple open-sided building, just a roof of sago palm supported on posts. We were met by a slight figure seated on a four-wheel all-terrain motor cycle. This was the medical superintendent, Dr Graham Tucker. With him was Barbara Fergusson, one of the team and a farmer from Salisbury, England. Her supporters had paid for the building materials of the 'hover-garage' we were to build. Barbara had arrived a few days earlier and was staying with the Tuckers.

Lurching along the 'road' in a four-wheel-drive utility truck, we peered through the steamed-up windows and rain for our first glimpse of the Balimo area. The red clay soil of the road was in an almost gelatinous state after several days of wet weather. Clinging tightly to any possible hold, we braced ourselves as the truck slithered from mudhole to mudhole. For two and a half miles (four kilometres) this is the only link between the airstrip and the health centre, which is the referral hospital for the whole of the Western Province of PNG. Desperately ill patients flown in for emergency treatment must be taken along this route, no matter what the conditions.

Refreshed by coffee and cakes provided by Graham Tucker's wife, Pat, we were ready to go off to inspect our home for the next two months or so. We could hardly believe our eyes. The rain had stopped and the sun was blazing down, illuminating the wonderful picture in front of us. Coconut palms on a steep bank framed a group of timber houses built on stilts and looking out over the lagoon. Two of these housed the principal and tutors from the nursing school, the other two were available for us. The raised floors gave shade beneath, as well as some protection from snakes. Inside, the houses were light and airy with rich-coloured timber floors and wonderful views. Dumping our rucksacks on the floor and looking around approvingly, we felt we too could make ourselves at home here. We had arrived.

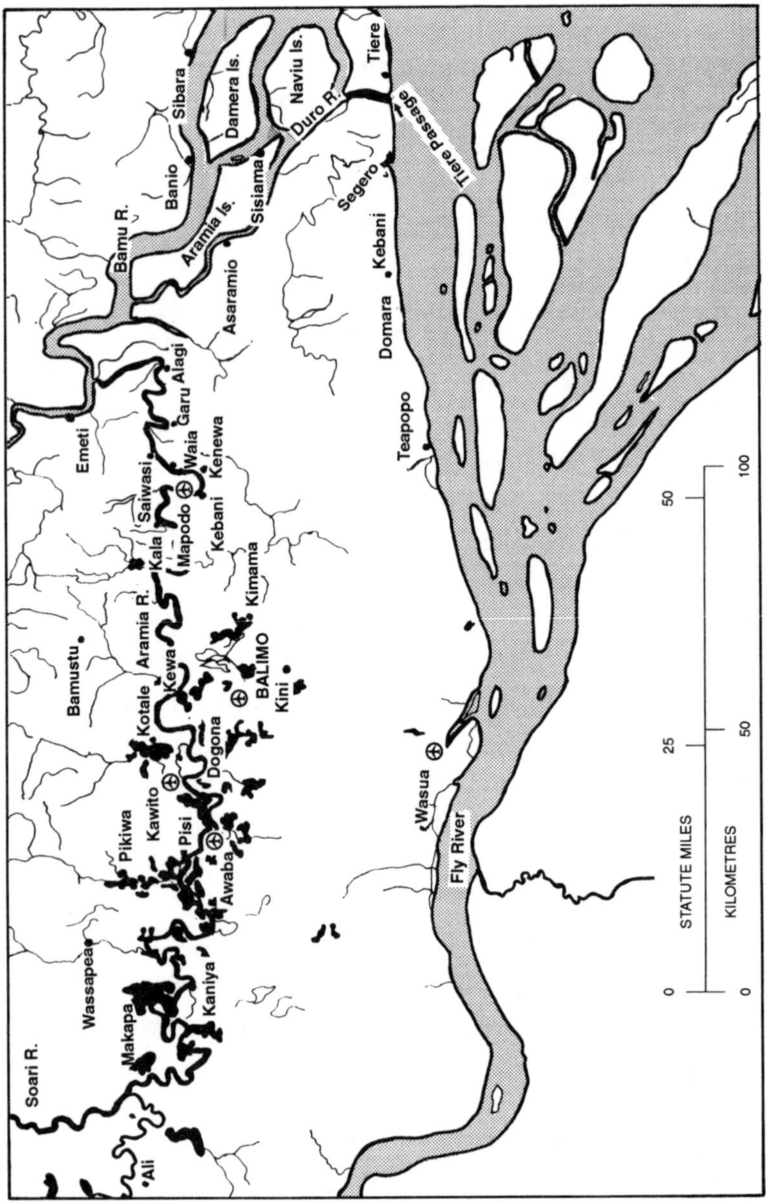
Soari R.
Ali
Makapa
Wassapea
Kaniya
Pikiwa
Kawito
Pisi
Awaba
Dogona
Kotale
Kewa
Bamustu
Aramia R.
BALIMO
Kini
Kimama
Kala
Mapodo
Kebani
Saiwasi
Waia
Kenewa
Emeti
Garu
Alagi
Asaramio
Bamu R.
Aramia Is.
Banio
Sisiama
Sibara
Damera Is.
Duro R.
Naviu Is.
Tiere
Tiere Passage
Segero
Kebani
Domara
Teapopo
Wasua
Fly River
STATUTE MILES
0
25
50
KILOMETRES
0
50
100

3

Spying and Supplying

EAGER TO GET TO grips with the work, Gordon and our two builders, Laurie and Andrew, with me in tow, went off to spy out the land. Pat Tucker had given us lunch and we had relaxed for a time enjoying the Tuckers' home and company. Now we were keen to be up and doing. Brian Black had arrived from Kawito on the mission station barge *Aramia*, with the first load of drums of gravel and food supplies from the container. The second planeload of team members had flown in and, after dumping their kit, had gone off with Brian to help unload the gravel. The action had started.

Laurie took the lead. He already knew his way around the area, and his long, lean legs carried him at a quick pace without giving any appearance of hurrying. For Gordon and me, it was our first opportunity to see the mission station and hospital, and we looked around with interest as we walked. We had seen something of the layout from the air as we came in but the rain had limited our view. My main impression, even in the rain, had been of a much more extensive area than I had imagined, yet it was dwarfed by the scale of the surrounding floodplain landscape.

Walking was to be our main means of getting about during our stay in Balimo as there were very few vehicles. It was certainly a good way to see the place. Leaving our new homes behind us, we walked away from the lagoon along the rutted clay 'road'. Across the open green space on our left we could see a long, low building built in the style characteristic of the area. The floor was raised above the ground on posts and the walls were of a dark-coloured timber. The roof of corrugated sheet metal extended to form a large shaded verandah and drained into a storage tank to catch the rainwater, the only source of drinking water. This was the Biula Church where services were held in Gogodala, the local language.

On our right was the mission workshop and next to it the home of Gauba, the mission handyman and driver. It was Gauba who had met us at the airport and driven us so skilfully along the quagmire of a track into the village. Further on, across another open green area as the 'road' veered to the right, were the long low buildings of the local school. Coconut palms abounded, offsetting the wide spaciousness and forming a backcloth to the buildings. We passed the Tuckers' house where we had lunched, and then two buildings where the students from the nursing school lived during their training. Unlike the Tuckers' house, these buildings had no space underneath. They were also enclosed by a tall wire fence to form a garden and recreation area. Other houses had no divisions around them.

Our track joined the track in from the airstrip and swung round to form the 'highway' past the hospital. Laurie took us on through the group of low buildings housing the hospital to the far end, where the noisy diesel generators were sited. With no company-maintained grid or mains supply for hundreds of miles, the hospital depends on these generators for electricity. Vital to the work of the hospital, they must run twenty-four hours a day. Two generators work in tandem so that if one fails the second cuts in automatically; failure of the electricity supply in the middle of a surgical operation could be fatal. Graham Tucker, who is also the hospital surgeon, often works on the maintenance of the generators himself, one of his many vital roles in keeping the hospital functioning. He is a man of many parts, and immensely practical.

One of our major tasks was to build a base where the two hovercraft could be housed and maintained. It needed to be close to the lagoon for launching of the craft, and to have ready access to the hospital for easy transfer of patients; an electricity supply and a means of getting fuel to the craft were also essential. We were looking for a site with all these features. Laurie, with his previous knowledge of the area, had already discussed some possibilities with Graham Tucker on the telephone. Beyond the generator shed and the adjoining workshops, the land falls away to the edge of the lagoon and in that area lay two potential sites.

'That's a possible,' said Laurie, his tall spare figure outlined against the sky as he stood on the edge of a bank looking down towards the lagoon. 'We'd have to clear away that ramshackle building down there,' he added, 'and take down those banana trees. We'd need to cut through the gardens on the edge of the lagoon, too.'

'Yeah, this site'd have some security, too,' said Andrew. 'The guys living in those huts alongside could keep an eye on it. And we could make a road down from behind the generator shed.'

'It's got to have a good run down to the lagoon,' said Gordon. 'Put it on the left where that old building is – that'd do it. The gradient's not bad, either.'

I stood there trying to disregard the lush vegetation as I

visualised the excavation that would be necessary. It certainly had 'capabilities' as Mr Lancelot Brown would have said.

It was a beautiful sight, with wonderful rich greens and a variety of forms in the vegetation nearby: sago and coconut palms, banana trees, grasses and sugar canes. The edge of the lagoon was formed by irregular banks of higher land, some jutting out like fingers of a hand spread wide into the water area. Between them the spits of land bounded large areas of grass-clogged lagoon. We looked out over one of these inlets across the tall water grass of the lagoon to the headland opposite, known as 'Government Point', with its tall radio masts and huts housing workers from the government station. Threading through the grass of the lagoon were a number of narrow channels of open water. Along these, members of the Gogodala people were paddling dugout canoes, their main means of transport over the vast area of the lagoon and river systems.

We were so close to the equator that the sun was almost directly overhead and burning down on us. With no shade and little cloud cover, the bank where we were standing was fully in the sun and already we were sweating profusely. It was certainly going to be demanding working in this humidity and in temperatures up to almost 100° F (38° C) in the shade. With relief we moved into the shade of the huts. Graham Tucker arrived and showed us the alternative site just a little distance away, but we quickly eliminated the second site in favour of the first. There was some doubt about the position of the boundary of the hospital land. Graham explained that he would have to consult the government representative, so we did not encroach on the adjoining communal lands which were jealously guarded by the Gogodalas. That would have to wait until the next morning.

The 'gravel party' had returned by the time we got back. Soon after their arrival at Balimo they were hard at work at the barge landing area near Government Point, loading the heavy drums of gravel onto a trailer for towing to our work site. Using a very basic lifting arm attached to the back of the tractor, the Gogodala driver hoisted the heavy drums one by one onto the trailer as the rest of the work party rolled them ashore from the barge. But starting up the steep slope from the water's edge, the trailer tipped over spilling a number of the drums, some into the water, and bending the side of the trailer too. This was not disastrous, but it needed a lot of extra work reloading the drums in the hot sticky atmosphere. We certainly had a lot to get used to.

We had to get used to living together as well. With only two loos and two showers, one of those a bucket shower, having up to twenty-four people in two houses was not going to be four-star accommodation. One house, known simply as Patterson's, had a large, open room and we decided this was where we would eat and hold meetings. Doing all our cooking in that house was also sensible. The other house, prosaically called Lagoon View, would function mainly as a dormitory. Rainwater was our only water supply, gathered from the tin roofs of the houses in large circular tanks. They had never been intended to serve our large numbers, so we would have to be very sparing in our water use and in the high temperatures that could pose some problems. Already we were conscious of the need to drink large quantities of water, and judging by our sweaty state, close living would not be any easier if we went without showering. We might just have to put up with each other at times. Below, on the edge of the lagoon, some Gogodala boys were romping in the water, and the pool looked very inviting. But the thought of the lurking dangers, possible conjunctivitis, ear infections, diarrhoea and even some obscure form of meningitis, was not at all attractive.

As it would be dark before seven, we had to get our sleeping arrangements sorted out between the two houses. The beds were an odd mixture of hefty slatted timber frames, some with foam mattresses, some without, and folding camp beds borrowed from the Australian Army. Rooms had to be allocated; who could share with whom? For the length of time we should be there some degree of compatibility was important. Snorers would certainly not be popular and local cultural susceptibilities also had to be taken into account. Single women were not allowed to share a house with single men, even if chaperoned by our married couple, Jenny and Gareth, yet it was apparently permissible for single women to stay in the same house as married men, even though none of the wives was present. This trust in married men only came out some weeks later when our two medical students Sarah and Aileen arrived with Ray (Rachel) Pinniger, our second woman doctor. Amanda Lee, for the present our only single young woman, stayed in an adjoining house with Jill Adams, one of the tutors from the nursing school. The next day she would be joined there by Rachel Grimmer. (Amanda is an accomplished linguist and no newcomer to Mike Cole's expeditions. She has led STEP teams and for a time worked as an assistant to Mike on administration of the STEP programme.)

With the comings and goings of team members and later the arrival of the four members of the film crew, deciding who could go where developed into a game of chequers, juggling between the various-sized rooms and acceptable groupings according to sex and marital status. In addition to the demands of leading the expedition Gordon had another role, that of billeting officer.

Disorganised as we were, it was good to be spared having to make our own evening meal. The Tuckers and others on the hospital staff had kindly invited us out for supper. Jenny, Gareth, Dick and I enjoyed a delicious meal which Debbra Roberts, principal of the nursing school, and Alison, one of the tutors, had laid on for us. It was not the sort of fare we had expected on our first night at Balimo.

After supper we had a briefing talk from Graham Tucker on various aspects of life at Balimo, things we would need to know for basic survival and to avoid any cultural gaffes. They were as varied as not stepping over people's legs as they sat on the floor in church (chairs were not used); not looking directly at a member of the opposite sex while talking to him or her, which could be tantamount to a sexual advance; never going out at night without a torch so we could be sure not to step on any of the three varieties of poisonous snake. Women were asked not to wear shorts or low-cut tops; this in a society where, until comparatively recently, women were clothed only from the waist down. Men were also told not to be surprised, but to take it as a sign of friendship, if a Gogodala man took our hand and stood holding it. This is apparently quite common in Gogodala society, and all part of getting to know people.

The many adjustments we had to make emphasised that we were in a very different culture and far from home. At the end of a long and busy day, when we had had so many new experiences, we were happy to spend some time together in quiet worship and thanksgiving before we went off to try to settle for the night in our new surroundings. It was at least a bit quieter here; Dick Bell's description of Port Moresby noises as 'frogs, dogs, crickets and cars' was not true in Balimo; here there were birds instead of cars.

Domestic matters had to be sorted out as a priority on our first full day. Arrangements don't just happen; someone has to work at them. For some months John Field had been planning for our catering needs. Schedules had been drawn up, draft menus considered and shopping lists prepared, even before most of us had given the matter a single thought. Many of the dried and tinned goods packed in the container had been on John's lists, including the dreaded 'compo' rations, donated to the Yangtze expedition as army rations that had passed their sell-by date four years earlier, in 1989. These became the butt of many jokes, yet were really quite impressive, despite their age. Maybe there is a moral in that! Now, surplus to Yangtze requirements, they had been bequeathed to us.

An army marches on its stomach, as Napoleon declared, and so we prepared for the day's work with breakfast at 7 am, followed by a brief time of prayer about the events of the day. Leaving John, Barbara and Amanda in charge of cleaning up and getting organised in the kitchen, Gordon split up the workforce. Gareth and Tim were to weld some reinforcement onto the lifting arm of the tractor to strengthen it for more heavy lifting; Laurie and Andrew, with Gordon, went to the building site to meet Graham in order to sort out boundaries, and the rest of us were delegated to move around equipment and beds between the two houses and to prepare for more of the team who were arriving from Moresby later in the day. Later we should be needed to unload another delivery of materials from the barge.

Help from the Gogodala people was at hand for clearance of the building site. Wielding long grass knives and machetes, several men from the hospital staff started to make short work of the job, under the appreciative eyes of the Gogodala audience. Banana trees, grass and undergrowth had to be cleared before a start could be made on rough setting out. The government representative had agreed that the site was entirely on hospital land so work could go ahead.

It had to go; the disused building was in the middle of the site selected for the new hovercraft base, leaning at an odd angle and looking ready to fall down. In fact, it was still very solid. Typical of the local construction, the timber frame was built of black palm and the roof covered with sago palm thatch. Like many of the living huts its floor was set high enough to allow a man to walk underneath it, providing a shaded and dry storage space beneath. The buildings for public use, the church, school and hospital, differed by having the floor set above ground but at about hip height. The wall covering had long been removed so it was easy to see that the floor was also of black palm, split into narrow widths and laid loose on the frame.

The hospital gang had a quick and effective demolition method which looked as if it had been used many times. A broad-shouldered, muscular young man came forward. He stood out from his companions because of his bright red waistcoat and broad-brimmed felt hat. Energetically he sawed three-quarters of the way through the uprights at knee height, while other men attached ropes round them, pushing the ropes high up the poles to roof level with the simple expedient of a long forked stick. With several men on each rope the tug of war began. They pulled gently at first, allowing the structure to sway back after each tug, then more strongly, building up momentum till the uprights were swaying like inverted pendulums. With a sharp crack, the whole building collapsed. The crash as it hit the ground bore witness to the solidity of the seemingly frail structure.

That was the easy part; now the wreckage had to be cleared. A few experimental heaves showed that it could not simply be pulled aside; it would have to be burned on the spot. A glowing ember from a nearby cooking fire was carried over in half a coconut shell and soon the tinder-dry thatch was blazing, adding to the increasing temperature as the sun climbed high. Until the fire died down, we could do nothing more there; we were free to go and help unload the barge.

The morning flight brought in four more of the team, including our two doctors Rachel Grimmer and Bill Gould. Our numbers had now built up to nineteen, although 'Bargemaster' Brian was still staying over at Kawito unloading and shipping gravel and stores. While we had sorted out our initial chaos, each new delivery from Brian served only to create more muddle as boxes and packages piled up everywhere. We still had mounds of tins and boxes of food to pack away, yet cartons of medical supplies were now coming in from Kawito as the goods packed in the container around the hovercraft were cleared. Until we got them out, the work of unloading and assembling the hovercraft could not start. Shortly before the container was packed at Gosport, Ray Pinniger had located a large quantity of surplus medical supplies at a Hampshire hospital that was closing down. Knowing that the Balimo hospital was always short of all kinds of medical goods, she had managed to secure a considerable quantity and had them packed on top of the hovercraft.

John and Amanda, with Barbara's help, were trying to organise lunch for us as the mound of incoming supplies took over most of the floor space. It was becoming difficult for anyone to move around.

'We've just got to get this lot sorted out,' Gordon said, his sense of order asserting itself.

'We're doing all we can,' replied John, looking harassed. 'It'd help if someone else would make themselves useful and put those tins in the storeroom.'

'Right, you chaps, get to work,' said Gordon. 'Put the compo rations, jam and marmalade in those packing cases. That'll get some of it out of the way.'

'And will someone hang up those nets of veg on the wall?' said Amanda. 'They're blocking the way to the storeroom.'

The confusion was becoming irritating, but with many willing hands around some order gradually emerged. However, the next day even more supplies would come, and the whole business would start again. We very much needed to find the best way of arranging ourselves and our stores so that we felt more at home and could concentrate on the job we had come to do. Necessary though it was, the organising seemed something of a distraction and we were impatient to get out and about, see something of the area and get into what we saw as the real task.

Borrowing the hospital dinghy and outboard, Gordon with Laurie at the helm took Brian back to Kawito rather than leave him to return on the slower barge. As they headed through the lagoon, Laurie was able to pass on his knowledge of the route to the Aramia River. The journey gave Gordon a chance to hear about Brian's progress in Port Moresby and at Kawito and to discuss the unloading and assembly of the hovercraft, which was the next important task. At Kawito Laurie was able to visit the sawmill and check when the timber he had ordered for the building would be ready for delivery. Leaving Brian for his final night at Kawito, the others arrived back at Balimo in time for our evening meal. By then I had done some preliminary setting out for site clearance and we had carted the new consignment of gravel drums from Government Point to our storage area by the hospital workshop.

So our second day drew to a close. Most of the team had arrived now and we were starting to settle into our new home. The travelling out had been tiring, but we were beginning to get over that. We still had to establish some routines for everyday living, catering duties, work and mealtimes, and to allocate responsibilities for the various aspects of our project, but at least we were now on the spot and able to get to grips with the work. This gave us some satisfaction and raised an air of expectancy.

The next day, Wednesday, the two Michaels, Cole and Pinkess, would arrive, making up the complete team for the first phase of our task. They had stayed in Port Moresby with Bruce Olsen to call on the British High Commissioner John Guy and various firms sponsoring us. They also had to set up local banking arrangements. Bruce's local knowledge and contacts were a great help. John Guy was very supportive and gave some financial help with the purchase of building supplies in PNG. He also agreed to attend the launching ceremony of the second hovercraft in Port Moresby in April. We hoped to have a government representative present, possibly the Prime Minister himself or the Minister for Health, and John Guy's support would be very helpful in achieving that. In early May, there was to be a formal handing over of the hovercraft service at Balimo and he promised to come to that too.

By our third day in Balimo, catering rosters had been drawn up and the unfortunate duty cooks had to be at work by 6.30 am preparing breakfast for the 'workers' by seven. That became the pattern so we could make a start on work for the day by 7.45 am. Until we had the hovercraft operational, many man hours would be spent travelling backwards and forwards between Balimo and Kawito. The sooner the craft were working, the better. While the distance is only about six miles (ten kilometres) as the crow flies (or perhaps in PNG terms as the whistling kite flies), the hospital dinghy with a load of four people could not make the journey following the winding watercourses in less than two hours. Packed away in the container were a Sea Rider semi-inflatable boat and outboard motor that would significantly reduce the journey time. We also needed it as a second support craft to the hovercraft and it was clearly a priority for unloading and assembly. Meanwhile, a canoe with outboard motor provided extra transport and seven of the team used it to go to Kawito, leaving the rest of us for duties around Balimo.

In those early days, using borrowed equipment, getting away on the water was never straightforward. Fuel was never in the right place, spark plugs needed cleaning or some other delay occurred. So it was some time before the Kawito party could leave. The delay allowed Jonathan Allan, as our official video man, time to film on the work site where a sago palm was about to be felled. Jenny, too, was there, taking still shots as the site clearance progressed. We were interested in the felling and processing of the sago palm, which provides the staple food of the area. Hearing the noises of knives hacking away at the trunk of the tree, our photographers assumed it was just preliminary clearance and that they had time to set up their equipment before the actual felling happened. With a loud crack, the tree was on its way down before they were ready. The pithy sago palm requires much less work to get it down than the more solid oak or beech trees we are used to. Watching the work was Larry, the Gogodala hospital manager, who told me that the sago palm reaches maturity for harvesting in only seven or eight years. This particular mature specimen would be processed by the women of the area within a day or so.

Tim and Andrew had fixed another attachment to the back of the tractor, a grader blade that would be used to pull the soil off the sloping site and excavate the clay beneath to give a level base for the building. First, an access road had to be cut down onto the site. Tim had not used this type of attachment before, but he was soon at ease with it, surprised by the versatility of this basic tool.

Any activity attracted an audience. Sometimes only children came, but at other times the men too would congregate on the bank above the site that formed a natural viewing gallery. No doubt it was unusual to see Westerners doing hard manual work in such heat and high humidity. The use of the tractor for grading and levelling was new to most of the Gogodalas, too. Such good progress was made on the new road that soon Tim was able to start stripping topsoil on the site below. The building site was far from level and there was a large quantity of clay to move. This clay would come in useful for making a bank along the side of the 'runway' up from the lagoon. On land a hovercraft can easily slide sideways on any cross-gradient and a bank helps keep it on track.

Easing themselves stiffly off the bottom of the narrow dugout canoe where they had been sitting for the last two hours, Gareth and Co. had no need to search Kawito for the container. It was sitting right in front of them, just clear of the water. That was as far as Brian and his helpers had been able to get it. Kawito had no sophisticated container handling equipment and the crane on the *Agutoi Chief* did not have the capacity to lift the combined weight of the steel container and its load off the deck. After much struggling, the box had been inched forward on rollers onto the shore until only a couple of yards still remained on the ship's lowered bow door. Three hours' work had been necessary to get it that far. Brian then resorted to the unorthodox and persuaded the captain to reverse his ship across the river away from the shore. The bow door dragged from under the end of the container, which dropped heavily onto the shore; there it had remained.

Most of the food and medical supplies had already been taken from the container. Now the Sea Rider and a second inflatable boat had to be moved to clear the way for unloading River Rover 401. At Gosport, a forklift truck had lifted the hovercraft up and forward onto the raised platform that had been built in the container. There was no such help to get it out at Kawito, but there was a great deal of manpower, a tractor and some steel beams that had been brought out in the container. As the tractor slowly towed the craft part way out of the container, the beams were placed under it. With many helpful Gogodalas holding each end of the beams the craft was simply lifted the rest of the way out of its box and placed on supporting pieces of timber on the sloping bank, ready for assembly. This was an impressive display of what can be done with sufficient manpower alone.

But the River Rover was a sorry sight. For ease of shipping the fan boxes and nose had been removed; the skirt had been taken off and the side decking dropped down. The cabin was stuffed with the fan boxes and other parts. The craft was like a self-assembly furniture kit, giving no hint of its final shape or purpose. To the curious crowd it must have looked very strange indeed, difficult to relate to the wonder craft they had been hearing about.

There was no shade over the work area and no easy way of providing any. All the assembly work had to be done in the full glare of the sun, which made it extremely demanding. Those working underneath the craft gained some relief from the shade, but they lost the benefit of any welcome breeze. And lying on your back for long periods with arms raised until they ache is not much fun; there was also the risk of legs sticking out from the shade, getting the full blast of strong ultra-violet rays on them. High-factor sun cream and sun block were much in demand, as were the water bottles we now carried with us everywhere. Without frequent litres of water, it was easy to become dehydrated quickly.

Gareth and Ben took the lead in the reassembly work. Ben Oliver in his work experience year had helped with the building of River Rover 401 and Gareth, an extremely practical and capable chap, had also done some work on it. Ben was a tall slim young man with an engaging grin. At times showing a maturity beyond his years, he also had a fun side to him and was popular at the nurses' meetings, where his guitar playing was much in demand. Gareth, twice Ben's age and immensely energetic, worked with earnest concentration, driving himself and always striving for high standards. He had originally trained as a mechanical engineer but later retrained as an electrical engineer. He also had experience in the building trades and so in practical matters was that rare combination, a genuine all-rounder. A gentle, kindly man, at times serious, he too had a lighter side and often surprised us with a high-pitched hoot of laughter. He and Ben formed quite a contrast, yet they worked together well and with mutual respect. Their experience was invaluable in the reassembly. Without that, the task would have been much more difficult, particularly as at that stage, by an oversight, we were without instruction manuals. There is no doubt that, even with manuals available, an engineer from HoverAid, the builders of the River Rover hovercraft, would have to oversee the reassembly for any other customer organisation in the developing world. Without the level of expertise that Ben and Gareth brought to the project, we should have been in grave difficulty.

HoverAid is a small charity producing specialised hovercraft for use in the developing world. It has been able to use the expeditions in some measure as a substitute for the huge programmes of research and development undertaken by multinational engineering concerns such as car manufacturers. This was to be an important aspect of the work in PNG, especially with River Rover 401, the first diesel-engined version used in tropical conditions. Without this development work, the pace at which these innovative small craft can be offered as a practical solution to medical transport problems in remote areas would inevitably be limited. It is a sobering thought that on such small privately funded ventures hangs the introduction of basic health care for so many people in the world.

Before the assembly crew arrived at Kawito, Brian had moved the barge over to the sawmill to take on board the first load of timber for the hover-garage, as it was now being called. With more supplies from the container, drums of diesel fuel and gravel, this was to be the 'Bargemaster's' last trip to Balimo where, finally, he would join the rest of us. He would no longer be the one-man advance party he had been at Port Moresby, Kawito and, initially, at Balimo. Brian was stocky in build and sturdy in character. He liked to get on with a job and not mess about and was not a man to suffer fools gladly. At times forthright, he was also considerate and very ready to help with anything he could turn his hand to. In the past he had been involved with merchant shipping and that, with his early role, had soon earned him the title of 'Bargemaster'.

Offloading Brian's barge on arrival at Government Point in Balimo proved to be a bit of a fiasco, or at least loading the trailer did. All we had to do was to put the timber and some of the fuel drums onto a trailer. It should have been simple, but somehow we managed to make a mess of it. The first lengths of timber came off the barge.

'Hey, some of these're longer than the trailer,' said Dick.

'Put the shorter ones in first,' said Tim.

Some of the watching Gogodala men came forward to lend a hand. They decided the longer lengths should stick out at the front, pointing up over the guardrail.

'That's no good,' said Tim. 'It'll foul the tractor when I turn.'

He knew what he was talking about, but they did not seem to agree, or else the message was not getting across. They carried on loading in the same way. I tried to minimise the effect by moving the long lengths into the centre.

'It'll still foul,' said Tim, shaking his head.

As it happened, this didn't matter. Some bright spark came up with the idea of dropping the tailboard and letting all the longer pieces stick out at the rear. Tim started driving the tractor up bank.

'Stop! Stop!' everyone yelled.

The whole load was bouncing backwards down the steeply sloping trailer. By the time Tim had stopped, three-quarters of the load was in the water, lying on the ground or sticking crazily up in the air over the back of the trailer.

There was nothing for it but to tow the trailer out from under and to start again, this time loading only the shorter lengths. With the tailboard up, everything stayed secure, and Tim and I went off to the workshop area to unload, followed by Andrew on a second tractor towing a load of fuel drums. The rest of the group carried the long timbers up the slope so we could load up on level ground, avoiding another fiasco.

Until we had everything we needed in one place, a great deal of time would have to be spent carting materials around. Apart from the building materials there were thirty-five drums of diesel fuel donated by BP for use in the hovercraft, and some drums of premix fuel donated by Shell for use in the outboard motors during the expedition. Everything had to be brought by barge from Kawito, landed at Government Point and carted to the work site. We seemed to be operating our own haulage company.

Mail arrived spasmodically at Balimo, coming on one of the three flights scheduled each week and going to the post office. Eventually it emerged from there and ours went to the hospital for our collection or sometimes Graham Tucker would bring it round himself. Bill Gould and Rachel Grimmer had been on a hospital ward round that morning and collected our first mail. It was seized on avidly when we all returned in the evening. One of the few to get a letter at that early stage was Amanda. To our amazement, she had a poll tax communication from her local council in the UK, correctly addressed to her at Balimo. We thought this was carrying the pursuit of poll tax dodgers too far and said so in no uncertain terms, only to have to apologise to Amanda and withdraw our rude remarks when it turned out to be that rare contradiction in terms a poll tax credit! How the council obtained her address remains a mystery.

Our numbers were down that evening. Although Brian was now with us, Gareth and Ben were staying overnight at Kawito so they could put in more time on the River Rover. The Tuckers at Kawito had kindly offered to put them up for the night. George Tucker ran the engineering workshop and sawmill there for the ECP (Evangelical Church of Papua New Guinea) and generously helped us on many occasions.

Loud chanting attracted our attention before breakfast next morning. Out on the lagoon was a splendid sight. A forty-foot long (twelve metre) dugout racing canoe was being driven through the water in great style by a crew of fifteen or so Gogodalas. The slim, low-sided dugout was brightly painted in a traditional tribal pattern of red, brown, black and white; its crew stood upright, wielding their long, broad-bladed paddles in unison, digging into the water with considerable force to propel the canoe forward at an impressive pace. The racing canoes have a special place in Gogodala culture, even in these Western-affected times. Carved from a single large trunk of carefully selected wood, they are skilfully shaped, often with an intricately carved prow in the shape of a tribal totem, and decorated in traditional tribal patterns. Stored ashore under their own sheltering roof of sago palm thatch, they are brought out only for races on ceremonial occasions or for practice; the races are fiercely contested. Seeing they had attracted attention, the crew put on a special show, coming closer inshore to be photographed and posing with raised paddles while intensifying their chants. The Gogodala people love to be photographed, especially the children, who run excitedly into grinning groups as soon as a camera is pointed even vaguely in their direction.

The canoe is the traditional form of transport in the whole of the Fly floodplain area. Children have small canoes from an early age in much the same way that Western children have bicycles, playing with them in the many pools around the edge of the grass-smothered lagoon. Women fish in their canoes from before sunrise each morning, and during the day canoes can always be seen coming and going through the water channels. Much of the paddling is done standing upright, balancing the slim craft agilely yet without obvious effort. It is hardly surprising that the Gogodalas have well-developed shoulder and arm muscles and walk with an easy grace. But the outboard motor is seen with increasing frequency. It extends the range of travel and speeds the transition from traditional food gathering to a cash economy. Once an outboard motor is used, even if only borrowed from a *wantok*, cash is needed for fuel.

The *wantok* (one talk) bond is a strong one, going far beyond the obligations of normal family relationships. It binds together tribal communities speaking the same language and stems from the past. Reflecting the difficult nature of the terrain, tribes were usually small groups rarely moving away from their own area, more than often treating a tribe only five miles (eight kilometres) away as strangers. There were more than 1000 separate tribal groupings in Papua New Guinea, speaking about 700 distinct languages (not just dialects). Suspicion and mistrust thrived on ignorance of others, even when living so relatively close. In a culture attributing every unexplained circumstance or mishap to spirit influences, evil or otherwise, mistrusted neighbouring tribes became the scapegoat for bad fortune. Local tribal warfare was often the result and has been a tradition of life in PNG for centuries. It still breaks out today, as two of our team were later to experience. The tribal warfare is evidence of the deeply entrenched 'payback' system and its demand for retribution, or at least for what is considered legitimate compensation. Against these strong influences allies are needed, and the *wantok* system provides that. A *wantok* can require any form of help from another, whether of goods, money or even warfare to exact payback revenge for the death of a relative. The obligation is mutual and honoured by strong tradition and so it is extremely powerful; members of the police force have even been known to go off to take part in a payback revenge killing and then return to their normal duties of keeping law and order. The influences are also at work in public life, so paralleling the distortions of corruption in other societies, making the task of honourable politicians and officials doubly difficult in this relatively new independent country. As we came to know each other and worked together, something of the *wantok* bond was growing within the team. We had come out acknowledging a common bond, but living closely together it was developing and growing in strength in our new environment. As pressure built up, no doubt the bond would be tested severely at times but certainly we were starting to see ourselves as *wantoks*.

4

Sago, Mossies, Ants and Such

Sago is unlikely ever to excite the gourmet even in its most refined form; not even when laced liberally with jam, as I remember it from schooldays. As served in Papua New Guinea, it is still less likely to inspire. Yet enormous effort goes into its preparation.

The sago palm felled in clearing the hovercraft slipway was not allowed to go to waste. The long, bare, spiky flower stems at the top, sticking up like the first bare branches of a stag-headed oak, showed it was ready for harvesting. Within two days men, women and children descended on it, and the process of turning the trunk into food started. Nor did the top go to waste. The long palm fronds were cut off at the base and the leaves were then stripped from the stem.

Both leaves and stems are used to make thatching panels for the sago thatch roofs so common in the area. The leaves are bent double over one of the stems, each leaf overlapping the edge of the previous one. Four or five leaves at a time are pinned together at the top and ends with sharpened wood slivers. The procedure is repeated until a panel is made up about five feet (one and a half metres) long and up to eighteen inches (half a metre) wide. Panels are laid on the roof from the eaves upwards, like very wide tiles, the stems uppermost. Each panel is placed to overlap the one below, gradually working towards the ridge until a thick, protective layer of the leaves covers the roof. Large quantities are required for even a moderate-sized roof, and the lengthy process has to be repeated periodically, as the life of a roof is no more than five years. The surplus stems are used upright to make partitions inside huts, forming dark-coloured bamboo-like screens.

Wielding their sharp machetes with powerful strokes, the men hack open lengths of the bark along the top of the trunk as it lies on the ground. A number of the women position themselves astride the trunk at intervals. Wielding narrow-bladed mattocks strongly, they hack their way into the tree, working in a slow steady rhythm. Meanwhile, children run around at play, sometimes scrambling along or across the tree trunk and often close to the swinging mattock blades. Four- or five-year-olds amuse themselves by brandishing long, sharp grass knives in imitation of their fathers' method of cutting grass or undergrowth. The knives swing from behind the right shoulder, swiftly arcing across the front of the body to wrap right around, almost to the back of the right shoulder again. The concentrated expression that accompanies this is usually replaced by a happy grin after several successful strokes.

As the women work the small chips of pithy wood they hack off pile up in front of them. Every so often they stop to gather the chips and stuff them into a long woven grass bag, then they go back to chipping. Once the grass bag is full, the women take it to the lagoon edge to dunk it in the water. The dripping bag is then lifted into a trough made from banana leaves and pummelled to saturate the pithy wood chips inside. Treading on the bag with bare feet washes the sago powder out as a milky liquid that is allowed to settle in the trough. Later the water is carefully drained off, leaving the damp sago behind to be dried out and stored as a meal. At best it will keep for three weeks before going mouldy, then the whole laborious business of gathering their staple food has to start all over again. It cannot be put off, no matter what the quantity gathered, for eating sago after the mould has started to grow can lead to an acute form of anaemia, which may be fatal.

Plantations of sago can be seen along the river banks, often with a small cultivated area close by that grows bananas and perhaps pumpkin. A family will tend the plantation and garden until the sago is all harvested, then move on to another plantation somewhere else within the tribal area, often travelling an hour or more by canoe away from their home. The plantations usually have a small, open-sided thatched shelter nearby to give some protection from sun and torrential rain.

Sago meal is served in only two ways. Mixed with water into a dough, it is cooked on an open griddle into a flat cake and eaten as a type of bread, otherwise it is mixed with pumpkin, coconut or fish, sometimes all together, wrapped in banana leaves and cooked in the fire. The resulting dark-green parcels of food have a squidgy feeling and a gelatinous texture in the mouth.

The quietly-spoken, gentle Gogodala people have little, yet generously they were always ready to share what they had whenever we visited them. They live on this food all the time, so it was interesting to share the experience with them.

Until the sago palm was completely out of the way, a start could not be made on forming the lower part of the runway down to the lagoon. The vegetation had to be cleared and the topsoil removed to give a firm, even surface for the hovercraft. A first attempt was made to even out some of the bumps and dips on the upper length of the runway, while the tractor was fitted up for similar work on the building site. Laurie had designed the building and drawn up plans months before; with Andrew he had made out material lists, too, and placed orders for what we required. But operating from a distance meant selecting the site had been impossible, as was following normal practice by having a preliminary site survey made before we arrived to do the work. So all planning decisions had to be taken on the spot while work was going ahead. Once the site had been cleared, we would get a better idea of the area available to us and how it related to the run-up from the lagoon.

Laurie had arranged for a surveying instrument known as a dumpy level to be flown in from Port Moresby so site levels could be taken but it did not arrive when expected. Fortunately he had with him a very simple gadget, no more than a tiny lightweight tube with liquid and an air bubble in it. With the line level, as it was called, clipped to a tightly stretched string line we were able to get some first indication of the amount of earth that had to be moved to make the area of the building level. We realised that much less excavation would be involved if the building were placed on the eastern side of the site rather than on the west, as originally intended. There could also be more direct access on that side for the delivery of fuel. It was still possible to have a smooth runway down to the lagoon from the eastern side of the site and the building would be well above any likely floodwater level during the rainy season. After consulting Graham and Gordon, it was settled we should build on the eastern side. Now that decision had been taken, a start could be made on setting out the precise size and shape of the building.

It was late when we got back to Patterson's that evening and we were surprised to find that the boat had not arrived back from Kawito. A party had gone over in the mission station dinghy that morning to help Gareth and Ben with the assembly work on the hovercraft, and they should have been back by then. This was only the second day the trip had been made and we had much to learn about the use of the boats on the lagoon. As darkness fell, our uncertainty mounted: what could have happened to them?

Martin Fairley, who was well used to electronic systems, tried to make contact with a VHF hand-held radio. We knew that one had been taken out on the boat. All Martin could get were raucous squawks of static and we were left doubting whether the boat crew had received any of his transmissions.

Inexperienced though we were at that time, we knew that the lagoon was not a good place to be stranded after dark. It really was black out there at night, and even with a torch it was not possible to see far. Until we got to know them better the many channels were confusing enough in the daylight; in the dark they would be impossible. Sitting low down near the water amongst the tall water grass, visibility was restricted, and in this very flat area very few landmarks could be seen even by day. In an uneasy atmosphere we started our meal. As we gave thanks for the food, we also prayed for the safety of those out in the boat.

It had been a hot and tiring day over at Kawito. Having stayed overnight Gareth and Ben were able to make an early start but there was still an enormous amount to do when the helpers for the day arrived from Balimo. They set to work with a will, refitting the fan boxes, drive belts, pulleys and fairings. Beneath the decking the diaphragm and skirt components had to be attached carefully in the correct sequence and position. Martin Healey concentrated on the separate task of putting together the Sea Rider semi-inflatable boat. The upper part of the hull had to be inflated and the engine control console fitted. As a keen and expert canoeist, Martin was experienced with boats. But even he came up against a snag:

'Hey, Gareth, have you seen the pack with the Sea Rider control cables?' he said.

'Wouldn't know 'em if I saw 'em, what're they like?' came Gareth's muffled voice from somewhere deep inside the back of the River Rover.

'Plastic bag with a couple of long black cables, I'd think,' said Martin. 'Must've been packed in the container with the rest of the Sea Rider kit in Gosport. They've got to be here somewhere.'

'Sorry, can't say I've come across them.'

Martin rummaged around in the back of the steel container, which by now was like an oven, standing in the blazing sun. There was still a layer of boxes under where the hovercraft had been packed. Gaps between the boxes could easily hide the slim package. Shuffling the boxes around was awkward and tiring, but they could not be moved out until the heavy metalwork for the garage had been unloaded.

'This is serious. I can't find them anywhere,' Martin announced. 'We've got to have them. There's no way we can control the choke and throttle from the driving position otherwise.'

'They must be there, you must have missed them,' said Ben.

'You find them, then!' retorted Martin.

Several overheated bodies scrabbling around without success in the ovenlike atmosphere of the container served only to increase the sense of frustration, coupled with the loss of time on the other tasks. The general consensus was that they should pack up, as they were wasting time. They would have to wait until the cables turned up while other things were being unpacked. In the meantime, the controls would have to be operated directly from the engine by a second crew member. It would not be the best way to travel or control the boat, but there was no alternative if it were to be brought into use. With the unplanned extra travel to Kawito the second boat was very much needed, and immediately.

The official launch of River Rover was planned for Saturday. There was still more assembly work to do and only one more day in which to do it. Gareth and Ben decided to stay overnight again, and they asked the rest of the crew to come back the following day, with a larger work party. Sea Rider was usable, despite the missing cables, so both boats were used for the return journey to Balimo. The new outboard on Sea Rider had yet to be run in, and so it could not be used at anything like full throttle, making it even more awkward to deal with the lack of the control cables. Jonathan, the only passenger, sat in the stern operating the short throttle lever on the side of the engine and struggling to hear Martin's shouted orders over the noise of the engine. Even with only two on board they could not make any faster speed than the following 'tin bath', as Martin disparagingly called the mission station aluminium dinghy, and the fuel consumption was higher than anticipated.

The engine spluttered to a stop. Martin and Jonathan had just entered the lagoon and were less than a quarter of an hour away from Balimo. The fuel tank was empty. It was not a calamity for there was a spare can of fuel on board, but in failing light and on the rocking boat, transferring the fuel was slow and messy work. Only a little way behind the Sea Rider, the 'tin bath' had the same problem. By the time both had been refuelled, darkness had fallen and the difficulty of making the final approach lay ahead.

With the darkness, the mosquitoes come. One moment there are none; the next there are hordes. Sometimes the menace is worse than others. Fortunately for the crews it was not too bad tonight. Just as well, for they had not expected to be back so late and had no protective creams with them, nor were they wearing long-sleeved shirts and long trousers. Their clothing, in fact, exposed a lot of flesh for the mossies to attack, and they are expert at finding it. The only thing the delayed travellers could do was to try to get back to base as quickly as possible. That would not be easy.

Mosquito control is expensive and difficult to effect. Control measures have been attempted in the past in various parts of PNG. They have failed and been abandoned in most places. The vast potential breeding ground of the whole swamp area is impossible to control, even if the money were available on the necessary scale, which it simply is not in this newly emerging nation that has so many demands on its limited resources. So the malaria carried by the mosquito is endemic in most parts of PNG and many of the population carry the malaria parasite. In addition to the general debilitating effects of repeated malaria attacks, the disease often leads to a potentially fatal condition. Malaria is best avoided, but few in PNG have that option.

Doctor Bill, as he was now being called, had prescribed anti-malaria pills for us some months before we left home and on his instruction we had been taking them for two weeks before our departure. Bill was a great asset on the team in so many ways: his wide medical and surgical experience in Nepal and elsewhere, his hovercraft expedition know-how from Peru and China, his cheerful even temperament, wisdom, sense of humour and engaging little chuckle endeared him to all the team members. 'Keep taking the pills' was one of Bill's catchphrases which caught on. He used it with a twinkle in his eye in all sorts of situations. And we did 'keep taking the pills' throughout the expedition.

The pills don't stop the mosquitoes biting. We had to take precautions to deter them, such as dabbing ourselves with citronella oil. Mosquito nets kept them at bay while we were sleeping. Even though our two temporary homes had wire gauze screens on all the windows and doors, some mosquitoes inevitably penetrated the defences. They could be heard droning around and carrying out their dive-bombing attacks. While the noise was low-pitched they were usually at a distance but as the pitch and intensity increased, we had to watch out – they were closing in for the attack. Sometimes the first indication of being a victim is the telltale spot of blood where the insect has been feeding.

Totally disorientated by now, Martin and Jonathan in Sea Rider, and Amanda and Graeme in the dinghy, had not a clue which way to go. They were not far from shore, but the blackness of a night unrelieved by a moon or by any other form of light masked that effectively. Setting off after refuelling, the boats nosed their way along whatever channel appeared. Each clump of tall grass looked exactly like the next; every water channel appeared the same. Progress was slow and what should have been a ten-minute journey stretched on. Several false leads turned out to be dead ends. Reversing out ran the propeller into the weeds and clogged it totally; the motor then had to be raised and the tangled mess cleared from around the propeller blades by fumbling in the dark. Eventually, a wider channel appeared and with quickening hope they followed it.

The telephoned message from Graham was a welcome interruption to supper: 'Good news – the boats have landed. Can you pick up the crews?' The boats had been spotted and someone had passed on a message. Tim abandoned his supper and taking our only transport, the tractor and trailer, set off with Laurie to collect the boat crews from Hospital Point, their departure point. But they weren't there; the channel that eventually led the boats to land had been the one to Government Point. There was confusion for a time but from his local knowledge Laurie decided the boats could well have gone in to Government Point. Ten minutes later Laurie and Tim were greeted with relief by the four waiting travellers.

But this was not a secure place in which to leave the boats overnight. Tim brought back Amanda, Graeme and Jonathan, while Laurie piloted the 'tin bath' around to Hospital Point, with Martin following in Sea Rider. There the boats would be under the care of Pilawa, one of the hospital staff who lived nearby. This meant yet another trip for Tim, to fetch the remaining crew and the engines. Then we were all secure together again. We gave thanks for that.

Mossies were not the only form of wild life we had to learn to live with. There were also the ants and the rats that seemed determined to share our food supply. While the ants were perhaps less worrying than the rats, they were certainly a great nuisance. Tiny black ants, far smaller than I am used to seeing at home, they could apparently get into everything. Attracted particularly by sweet things, they were nevertheless not too choosy. Nothing was safe from them. The hospital's egalitarian tearoom was close to the building site and, despite our grimy work clothes, we were made welcome there along with the nurses, surgeons, health orderlies and others for a short break any morning we cared to stop by. It was a welcome respite from the sun and another opportunity to replace some lost fluid. Sitting there one morning with Andrew and Laurie I was amazed by Andrew's antics with a packet of biscuits. The large dry beef crackers were a favourite with the male Gogodala hospital staff and our two Queenslanders had clearly acquired a taste for them during their previous stay. Stripping off the sealed cellophane wrapping, Andrew picked out one of the large biscuits and holding it upright, absently tapped it sharply several times on the table. A whole horde of tiny black ants came tumbling out and scurried across the table. Undaunted, Andrew broke off a sizeable chunk and popped it in his mouth. Seeing my amazement, or perhaps horror, Andrew laughed: 'Only a bit more protein!' He crunched on in evident enjoyment. He seemed to stay quite healthy despite, or perhaps because of, the extra protein.

The rats were a different matter. No one was prepared to tolerate them. They first made their presence known by practising rugby tackles in the roof space, or at least that was what it sounded like. The roof construction was only light, with fibreboard linings to the ceilings. It acted like a drum skin and noises above reverberated loudly. The scamperings and thumps disturbed the lighter sleepers and the thought that the rats might not confine their activities to the roof space was not a comforting one. Soon we found evidence that they had been visiting the kitchen. This had to stop. A wire trap was found and used with some success, although we never did stop the rugby entirely.

The species of spider that lived in the dry soil beneath the house was not threatening to us but interesting to observe. In the dust we found shallow depressions about two feet (sixty centimetres) across. Spaced out over the depressions were little hollows. Unsuspecting insects foolish enough to walk across or close to one of these small hollows disappeared in a swift flurry of dust, the victims of tiny spiders that burrowed into the dust and lay concealed in the hollows patiently waiting for dinner to walk by, which it did with surprising regularity. Leaping up, the spiders seized the poor victim and quickly dropped back out of sight into their holes presumably to await the next course. Mischievously, to see what would happen, we smoothed the dust lightly over a whole colony of the holes. After a short time, while they were no doubt muttering imprecations at this unnecessary work, puffs of dust spouted up from the ground, as with a great deal of vigour the spiders excavated their traps again. It's a hard world, the insect one.

One of the threats flying insects must face is the gecko. This fascinating creature was a friend as far as we were concerned, but no insect could treat it as that. Our variety of this terrestrial lizard was quite small, no more than six inches (fifteen centimetres) long. Both indoors and out, they performed a useful service in seeking to keep down the flying insect population. Judging by the remaining insect numbers, the place could have supported many, many more geckoes. They seemed to establish territories on the wire gauze fly screens on the outside of the louvred windows, about five or six per panel. Any intrepid trespasser was seen off the territory with a threatening rush similar to the speedy dive the geckoes made to gobble up an unwary flying insect. Their ability to cling to vertical surfaces or to run upside down across the ceiling was impressive. The adhesive pads on their tiny, distinctly formed digits are very effective. For such a tiny thing the gecko can make a surprising amount of noise, so much that I did not relate it to them for quite a while. The indoor geckoes would punctuate our conversations with what seemed like little noises of exasperation. It was hard not to look around the team to see who was disapproving, as the sharp 'tchk, tchk, tchk' noise sounded clearly from time to time.

Noise was the way in which others of our neighbours made their presence known, particularly at night. As I live in the depths of Herefordshire farming land, the noises of the 'quiet' countryside are very familiar to me. But they are soft and gentle compared with the noises of the lagoon. The lower notes are provided by the frogs, spanning a wide range from deep bass rasping notes to sharp little trebles. Together, and multiplied many times over, the level of sound is considerable. The higher pitched accompaniment comes from the cicadas, whose monotonous, continuous noise provides a steady background to the intermittent croaks of the frogs. It's the chaps who are to blame, apparently. The male cicada has a couple of drumlike organs (of the medical not the musical kind) in his abdomen which for some strange reason he vibrates continually to produce a high-pitched drone. The frogs and the cicadas seem to be very time-conscious; every evening, without fail, they switch on just before seven as darkness is falling and continue without pause into the early hours of the morning. I am not sure at what time they switched off as I managed to get some sleep despite their efforts, but certainly by about three in the morning it was much quieter. Maybe by then they were just exhausted.

The frogs were also responsible for many a raised pulse rate. We had been warned by Graham Tucker not to go out at night without a torch, so we could keep a wary eye out for poisonous snakes. We used up many torch batteries. As we walked across the grass areas around the houses at night, we would anxiously swing the torch backwards and forwards so the beam crossed our path. A quick movement on the periphery of the light could certainly cause a momentary slowing of the pace, if not a sharp jump in the opposite direction. Usually it was a frog hopping slowly on itsway, unaware that it had almost caused heart failure. If, as frequently was the case, it was necessary for one of us to make a phone call or use the radio, we would have to walk to the Tuckers' house a few minutes away through the blackness. On the duckboard at the foot of the stairs to the front door, there was always a group of five or six frogs enjoying the glare of their outside light in much the way we would bask in the sunlight.

We had ample incentive not to wander around at night when staying out in the villages or on the river, unless it was absolutely imperative. One night Debbie, the principal of the nursing school, came over with some things she wanted Mike Cole to take downriver. Debbie had only been gone for a few minutes when she returned and asked with a glint in her eye.

'Do you want to see what I met on the way home?' she asked.

Only when we spotted the three-foot-long grass knife in her hand did we suspect that her question was not quite as innocent as it appeared. Curiosity overcame our doubts and four of us followed her out. There in the beam of her torch was a five-foot-long (one-and-a-half metre) taipan, one of PNG's three varieties of deadly snake. We eyed it nervously from a distance. Debbie laughed.

'It's all right,' she said. 'I've killed it.'

The snake was stretched out on the grass where Debbie had struck with her long knife. She told us that the taipan had slithered into the narrow beam of her torch as she crossed the grass area between the houses. Instead of taking to her heels and locking herself safely indoors, as I am sure many of us would have done, the cherubic, mild-looking Debbie had coolly gone in, got her knife and attacked the snake, even though its bite can kill. The next day, following the violence of her act the night before, she was lecturing her students on the finer points of the gentle care of their patients.

Despite these terrors, we were keen to go further afield. Most of us had not left Balimo and our first Friday offered that opportunity. As many as possible of the team were to join Gareth and Ben at Kawito to help finish the assembly of River Rover 401. On Saturday it was scheduled to make its first appearance at Balimo, and anticipation was mounting among the Gogodalas. We couldn't disappoint them, so a big push was needed. With an effort it might be possible to have a test launch at Kawito later in the day to make sure the hovercraft was up to scratch. Laurie and Andrew were to carry on working on the building site with Brian Black helping, while Jenny offered to stay home, look after the houses and prepare the evening meal.

Sea Rider could not cope with a load of more than four; that left eleven of us needing transport. A Gogodala dugout canoe fitted with an outboard motor was hired with a crew of two and arrived in the creek below Patterson's, our main house, about 8 am to pick us up. Getting in was an experience in itself and did nothing to reassure us about the stability of the craft. Teetering from side to side, we boarded at the bow and made our unsteady way down the canoe. The bow was the only part on solid ground and the canoe rocked alarmingly at the slightest movement. Then, unsteadily, we had to turn around and sit down on some rough duckboards in the narrow bottom of the canoe, packing our bags in between us. Finally we were all on board and we were pushed off into the lagoon.

The canoe was surprisingly stable. Sitting in the bottom, we provided good ballast; I certainly would not have given much for our chances standing up. Carved, or rather hacked, out of a single tree trunk, the canoe sides were a few centimetres thick, the bottom, I assumed, being thicker to form a sort of keel weight. The wood was very hard and smooth. The top opening was narrow, barely more than half the width of the log, then the width inside increased to almost the full span of the log at the centre and reduced again to the bottom. As a result there was very little room to spare at the rim just below shoulder height.

Travelling out through the lagoon so close to water level gave a good view of the aquatic plants, grasses three feet (a metre) or more above sea level, and several types of water lily with mauve or white flowers. Wading birds about the size of a redshank with long spindly legs skipped lightly from lily leaf to lily leaf, and overhead sea eagles wheeled, occasionally plunging down with barely a splash to rise with a fish between their claws. The channels in the lagoon twisted around through the grasses, joining up with others and dividing off many times. Although we kept a wary eye out for crocodiles, we did not spot any. They are still around but much reduced in number due to hunting, mainly for their meat.

As we rounded a bend another canoe would appear, sometimes with a lone woman sitting fishing with line or net; others would carry families with father and mother both standing paddling easily and gracefully. Care was always taken that the wash from the outboard did not rock or swamp another canoe, particularly those with little freeboard. Almost half an hour passed as we travelled at a moderate pace, before we came to the Aramia River itself; a small tributary of the river formed the outlet from the lagoon.

The Aramia is wide in places; in the Balimo-to-Kawito section more than one hundred and thirty-one feet (forty metres) across.

As we travelled, first the sun would be on one side, next on the other as the river meandered in broad loops, turning around in a bewildering way. Occasionally we passed small settlements set on high ground, well above the present low water levels. Families were fishing from the bank or canoes, often close to sago plantations and small gardens with banana trees. They waved greetings as we passed. In a couple of places new dugout canoes were being made, the bright newly carved wood contrasting starkly with the dark weathered wood of our own.

It was more than two hours before we could ease our cramped limbs on arriving at Kawito. We had expected to be overtaken by Sea Rider but with four people on board and the engine being run in, the boat was unable to get up much speed. It arrived some time after our canoe, to much leg-pulling, of course.

A great deal of work still needed to be done on assembling the hovercraft and soon everyone was over, under and around it like a swarm of ants. Working in twos and threes on various aspects of the assembly, the work mainly involved screwing and bolting parts together. It was not difficult but the trick, of course, was to get everything assembled in the right order. Gareth was general overseer, while trying to deal with the more complex parts himself. There was a continuous chorus of, 'Gareth, how should this fit?', 'Gareth, what goes here?', punctuated from time to time by similar appeals to young Ben who had worked on the building of the craft with Steve Moody. There were also constant appeals for tools: 'Is there an eight-millimetre socket free?', 'Anyone got a large screwdriver?', and so on, despite the fact that several sets of tools were in circulation. Feet protruded from under the craft in many places and bodies were contorted into all sorts of shapes to reach seemingly inaccessible areas. Why is it that engineers, who must spend much of their time doing this sort of thing, seem to revel in creating impossible positions in which it is essential to place a tiny nut or screw?

One pair of protruding feet belonged to Bill Gould, our surgeon. He was lying on his back underneath the decking, fixing the upper part of the hovercraft skirt in position. Standing above him, two others were feeding parts and tools to him on his instructions, or locking a spanner on the outer end of the bolt he was fixing. 'Bolt,' he demanded, and one was placed in his open palm which came out from under the craft. 'Washer,' – that too was placed in his hand. 'Nut ... spanner ... thank you, sister!' Clearly this was just another operation to Bill.

Amanda acquired yet another nickname after she managed, despite warnings, to put so much strength into her work that she sheared the small bolt she was tightening. 'Dear Amanda' became 'Shear Amanda' adding to the 'cute Pom' label she had acquired in Port Moresby from the Olsen family.

Panels were bolted on, skirt sections and retaining straps assembled, pipes fitted and a thousand and one other things done. It was just as well we had such a large workforce. Barbara Ferguson played her part in a number of ways but finished up with the thankless yet important task of scraping mastic sealant off the nose section prior to its reassembly. Gareth gave me the job of drilling out the various boltholes for the nose so the refitting job would be done more easily than the dismantling. While all this was going on logos of various sponsoring organisations were plastered all over the craft ready for later photography.

All the work was carried on under the watchful eye of a massed crowd of Gogodala. They were on the verandahs of some buildings on the slope above, and on the adjoining higher ground which formed a natural grandstand for them. They took a keen but fairly silent interest in all we were doing. We must have seemed a strange crowd to them, although with their tribal culture the concept of working together on tasks must have been very familiar to them.

Despite the large workforce, we would clearly not have River Rover launched that afternoon before we left to return to Balimo. Gareth and Ben stayed for a third night to do some more work and look after the craft and stores. George and Lorraine Tucker were kindly feeding and housing the two of them all this time. They also gave us the freedom of their house for topping up water containers, washing and making up sandwiches, which Rachel and Amanda did for us. The Tuckers, like all the ECP staff we met, did everything they could to help us, and we were very grateful for their unstinting support.

John Field recovered his Zodiac inflatable and its outboard motor from the container. Keen to use it and unworried by a continuous leak of air from the right-hand side of the boat, he and Dick decided to return in it to Balimo. Dick was going to pump air into the Zodiac during the journey in an attempt to keep it inflated. They set out first so that if they got into trouble the following canoe and Sea Rider, rather than the lurking crocodiles, could help them out. We set off in the canoe and had another enjoyable, although cramped, trip. I was sitting nearer the bow on the return journey and a combination of wind and bow wave provided a refreshing spray. At one point the canoe overtook the leaking Zodiac. Dick was bent double, pumping away furiously in the bottom of the craft. Despite that, they seemed not to need rescue, so we carried on. Both the other boats arrived after the canoe. Unfortunately Sea Rider took the wrong channel on the way into Mission Point, fouling and damaging a local fisherman's net. Michael Pinkess, with his insurance broking experience, was duly appointed compensation officer to deal with the clearly admitted claim, Laurie apparently knowing the man involved. Laurie's local knowledge was proving invaluable again.

So, tired but cheered by the thought of bringing the hovercraft to Balimo the next day, we enjoyed Jenny's cooking, caught up on the building site team's efforts and felt satisfied with the day's work. With all that behind us, even the frogs, dogs and crickets were unlikely to keep us awake for long.

5

The Grand Arrival

THIS WAS IT. The big day the local community had been waiting for; the day when the first of the much-talked-about, wonderful new machines was to arrive at Balimo. The Gogodalas had been hearing about the hovercraft for some time now and there was an air of eager anticipation. A cutting from the Port Moresby *Post Courier* pinned to the hospital notice board for some weeks, carried a report about the hovercraft and a picture of it taken in England. Now everyone would be able to see and hear the real thing.

So many of the Balimo people had benefited from the hospital, had worked there, or were related to someone who did that almost anything to do with the hospital was of interest. They knew about the effective work of the health patrols in the villages along the river system. They knew of the many times that the Mission Aviation Fellowship (MAF) had been called to fly in a patient in a serious condition; sometimes these patients should have received earlier treatment, but the cost of a flight, even at MAF rates, had deterred an earlier call-out, at times for far too long.

Now the hospital was to be given these splendid new craft. They would speed up the medical patrols and make it possible to bring in emergency cases more cheaply. It was a day for celebration and everyone looked forward to it.

The work of the Balimo Health Centre extends far beyond the lagoon. It is the referral hospital for the whole of the Western Province of Papua New Guinea, which has a population of more than 100,000. In addition to the inpatient and outpatient services it provides a basic health care programme spanning the whole southern Fly area. Six health sub-centres and fourteen aid posts are provided throughout the area and there is a vigorous health care programme in the village community schools.

The scale of the work is impressive, there were more than 1700 admissions in 1992, 54,000 outpatient attendances, 4500 immunisations, 2400 dental treatments and an extensive laboratory service. The health sub-centres account for another 90,000 outpatient attendances and a similar number of immunisations, and almost as many dental treatments as at Balimo are provided during visits to community schools.

These services are provided by the hospital as an ECP Health Agency institution. Some help is received in the form of an annual grant from the government, but the level of funding is still not being met in full; the provincial government agreed to pay return air fares for patients who paid for their own incoming flights, but accounts for those fares have not been settled. At Balimo Francis Koimanrea, the Minister for Health for Papua New Guinea, said, 'The government does not have the money and resources to do the job. The churches have shown that they are committed to improving health services for the people and they have done the job better than the government.'

Yet this valuable service is delicately balanced and teeters on the brink of insolvency. Unless government funding is given to the full agreed level, the present services are in jeopardy, and without the hovercraft there would be no possibility of extension to villages just beyond the present range. The contrasts in health standards in those unreached villages is dramatic. Major advances can be made simply by introducing a basic health care programme. No wonder staff and villagers alike were excited at the arrival of the hovercraft, which would do just that. The excitement was not just confined to the Gogodalas. For the team, too, this was an exciting day. For months we had been preparing for it, thinking about it, talking and writing about it, planning for it, working towards it. Now we had finally arrived at the first objective; bringing the hovercraft to Balimo. Over breakfast there was a holiday atmosphere; even the slow starters showed some animation and the banter was even more lively than usual.

Government Point had been specially tidied up for the occasion and an area roped off for beaching the hovercraft. The arrival was scheduled for 2 pm, when there was to be an official welcome and reception by Graham Tucker. Saturday was the first possible day the hovercraft could be ready, but it had also been chosen because people would be free to come along to the biggest happening at Balimo for a long time. News had spread far and wide, and people were coming in by canoe from villages up and down the Aramia and around the lagoons, so a large crowd was expected to witness the great event. Unconfirmed rumour, or possibly just speculation, suggested that the racing canoe practice we had seen one morning had been in preparation for a celebration in traditional style.

Over at Kawito there were still things to do. The two Martins had left early in Sea Rider with Jonathan, whose job was to capture the launch at Kawito on video film and then immediately dash back to Balimo to be in place to film the arrival. Until the production team for the official video arrived in a few weeks' time Jonathan was responsible for capturing significant moments on film, for the video and for our own records. He and the two Martins would also be able to give Gareth and Ben some help on any last-minute jobs.

Mike Cole was to have the privilege of launching River Rover and driving it to Balimo. That seemed highly appropriate as he had been working towards this moment for several years. Gordon Goodman, the field leader of the expedition in PNG, was to travel with him, as were Dick Bell and Bill Gould, veterans of the China expedition with Mike. They left Balimo mid-morning, giving the engineers time to complete the last-minute checks before they took over as the official launching party.

Most of the remainder of the team had time to relax. However, poor Laurie was unable to do so, as he was the first victim of the dreaded 'Balimo tum'. Ironically, he had been the one to warn us of it. 'It's not a question of whether you get it,' he had predicted, 'but when.' He said he was feeling 'real crook' and he looked it. At first malaria was suspected, but tests soon ruled that out. Leaving him suffering, Andrew, Brian and I went to the building site, as we had some work to finish so the hovercraft could be brought around there after the ceremony. First Andrew had to help get the hospital dinghy organised for the launching party to use, so there was a little time in hand before we could start work. I wandered off into the village to take some photos on the way over to the site.

As I neared the hospital, people were streaming towards it and by the time I got there a large crowd had gathered, possibly a hundred or so men, women, and children. They were standing in front of one of the huts beside the road, silently directing their gaze towards the open verandah. As I moved closer, I saw a group of nurses kneeling on the verandah with an oxygen cylinder trolley by them. It looked like a training exercise so I took a photo for the record. As I moved a little nearer, the group of nurses parted and moved the oxygen cylinders to one side. A man was lying on the verandah. This was no exercise; the man started to groan, clearly in some distress. One of the nurses looked around her, momentarily at a loss. There was nothing I could do to help with experts on hand, so I moved on. Not until the evening did I learn that a relatively young man, suffering from a rheumatoid heart condition, had been sitting out on the verandah in the sun when he had suddenly collapsed. Shortly after I left, he died. This was the second death at the hospital that day; earlier a woman had died in one of the wards. It was a distressing day for the staff, one that brought home to me the desperate need for medical services here. With all the problems they face, these dedicated people need and deserve all the help the hovercraft can bring them.

Then unaware of the real drama I had left behind, I sat quietly in the shade waiting — it was going to be a very hot day. Andrew must have been delayed. I learned the reason when Gordon and Bill appeared, walking up from Hospital Point. They should have been well on their way to Kawito by then. As seemed to be the pattern, there was trouble with the outboard motor on the borrowed hospital dinghy. A part had to be cannibalised from John Field's outboard motor to effect a repair before they could get off, and there was no fuel with the boat. Our own fuel stocks had not yet been organised properly, so there would be a further delay. It would be tight keeping to the schedule now. Finally Andrew got them on their way.

Good progress had been made on the site but some final

levelling was still needed. The dumpy level had eventually been flown in the day before, so at last we could finish the first phase of the excavation. Andrew set to work on the tractor fitted with the grader blade while, aided by Brian holding a measuring staff, I used the level to keep a check on the amount of clay Andrew needed to scrape off. Time was getting short if the work was to be completed and the site left spick and span, ready for the grand arrival later in the day.

We were late back for lunch and it was a rush to get cleaned up and be ready in time. The first sign of trouble came as we were about to leave. A message came down from the Tuckers' that the arrival had been put back to 3 pm. This was not surprising, we reasoned, in view of the delays earlier in the day, especially if a load of four had slowed down the 'tin bath'.

A colourful sight greeted us as we walked down the road later. Bright sun umbrellas were much in evidence amongst the large number of people streaming down. This was clearly a popular event; only as we walked further down the road did we realise that the hovercraft arrival was not the sole reason for the gathering crowd. The competing attraction was the local rugby match. Rugby is very popular in PNG. We found the ground was on our route and with a little time in hand, we paused to see some of the game. It was on a full-sized pitch with regulation posts and had a small grandstand. The game was being played with a great deal of gusto, if not finesse. Tackles often seemed to involve heaving the ball holder totally off the ground and swinging him around until he gave up possession. And all this under a blazing sun! Tearing ourselves away, we continued down to the landing point.

It was a natural amphitheatre with a steep ramp down to the water. It gave a good view out over the grass-smothered lagoon framed by headlands to right and left with their huts and coconut palms silhouetted against the brilliant blue of the sky. Already many people had gathered at vantage points on the banks to witness the great event. Some had come by canoe from riverside villages many miles away and there was a holiday atmosphere. The sun shone on the brightly coloured clothing in the crowd and the rainbow-panelled umbrellas used as sunshades. A number of the men were using umbrellas to shade young babies. Despite the male domination of this society, it is not unusual to see a Gogodala man holding a baby. They often mind the children while the women are out fishing on the lagoon or perhaps hacking away gathering their next supply of sago meal. Fathers may even be seen out in the open holding a young child by one arm while sponging it down over a bowl of water.

There was a general air of anticipation, and our arrival caused a stir of interest. We were readily identifiable by our white skins and our team shirts displaying the expedition logo, which combines a hovercraft and the bird of paradise, the national symbol of Papua New Guinea. The hovercraft would first come into sight around the headland of Hospital Point away to our right, then come sweeping around the arc of the main channel to beach immediately below us. As we selected telephoto lenses ready for the first distant sighting, the young boys were particularly interested in our cameras. They crowded in ever closer, perhaps hoping to be photographed. Brian Black caused some excitement and lots of 'oohs' and 'ahs' when he went down below the bank and, much to their delight, he turned his video camera on the crowd above. If that excited them, we thought they would go wild when they saw the hovercraft.

Sudden shouts of excitement and little boys jumping up and

down in the crowd to our right had us lifting our cameras to the ready, thinking that they had seen the hovercraft appearing. It turned out to be a false alarm. Just after that Ian Wiley, an Australian revisiting Balimo where he had previously worked, appeared at our elbows. We had passed Ian on the road on our way down. Quietly he said,

'Graham Tucker's had a radio message. The hovercraft's going to be an hour late. They've got it on the water but can't get enough lift.'

'Not enough lift?' I was puzzled. 'What's the problem?'

'Don't know, but they're definitely going to be late,' said Ian.

'This lot's not going to like that,' said Brian looking round at the crowd. 'Hanging around for another hour, they've been here ages already. How're they going to react when they hear the news?'

It was a fair point. Hemmed in as we were, the frustration of an already excited crowd could be a force to be reckoned with. It was not a comfortable thought.

Immediately, too, long-held doubts came flooding back. Was the craft really underpowered? Originally some had not been convinced that the diesel unit of the Mk IV would give the same power as the high-revving petrol engine of the Mk III. The successful trials at Hoddesden the previous November, when both types had been shown to perform equally well, had done much to dispel these doubts, but they had not been entirely removed.

Quickly these concerns were swept away again by thoughts of how this excited crowd would react when they heard the news, and whether we could stand around waiting for another hour or more in the broiling sun. The alternative was to sidle nonchalantly away, hoping no one would notice, and face the long walk back in the heat, only to return later when we knew for sure the craft was

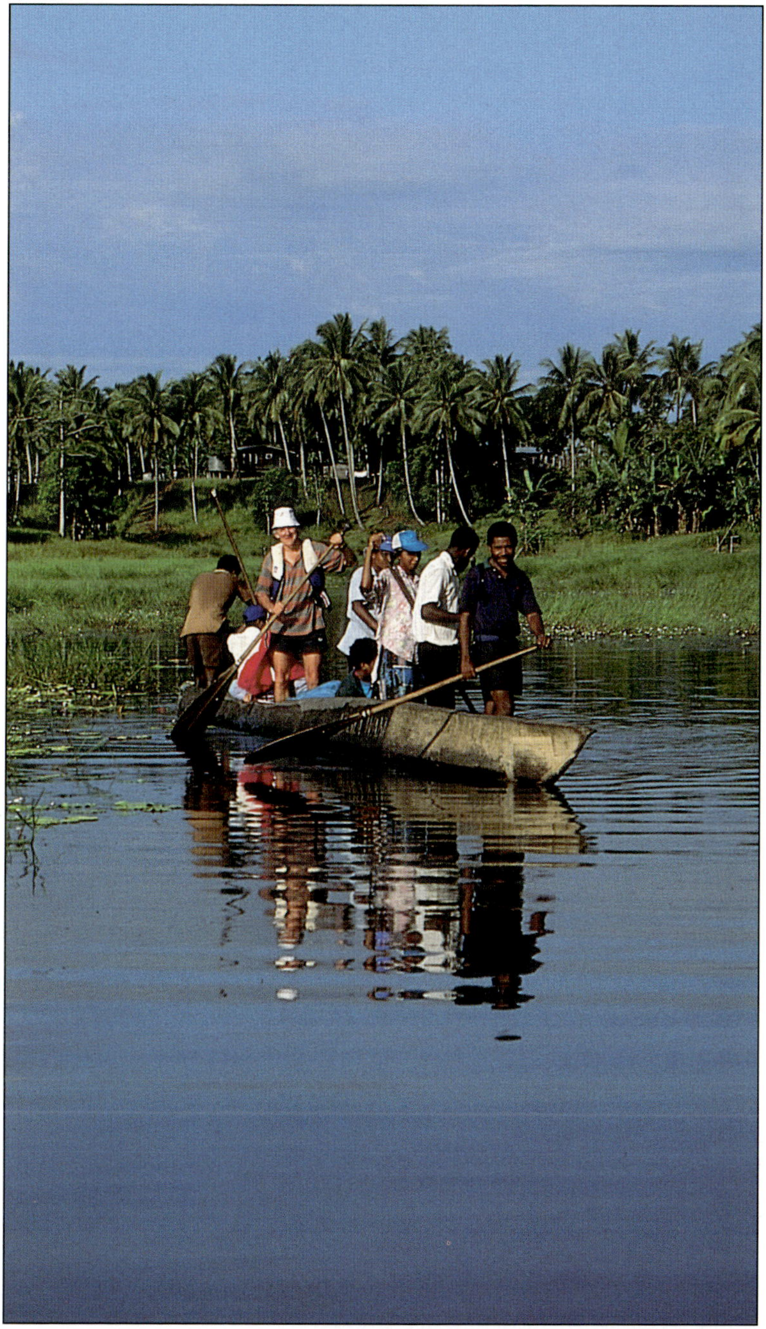

Traditional patrol

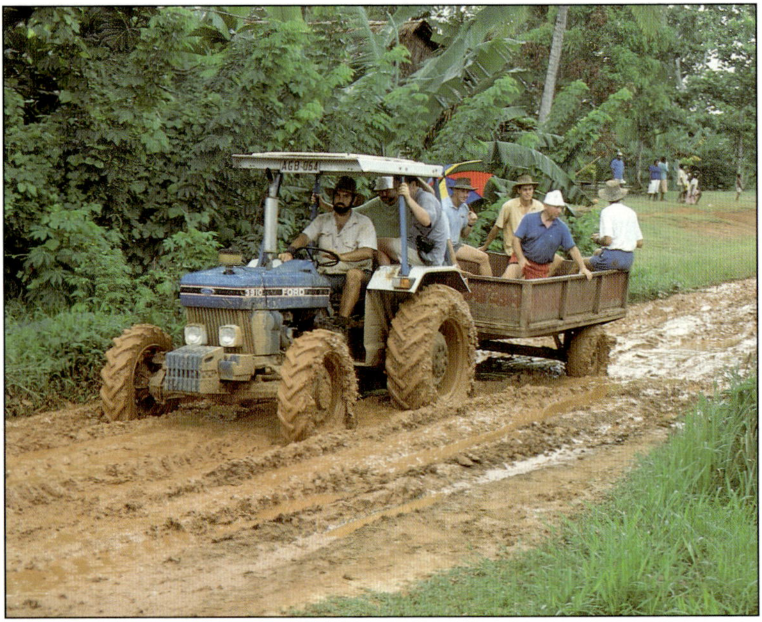

Above: Andrew Schache driving the airport bus to Balimo airport
Below: First hovercraft medical patrol
Right: Conquering the lagoon

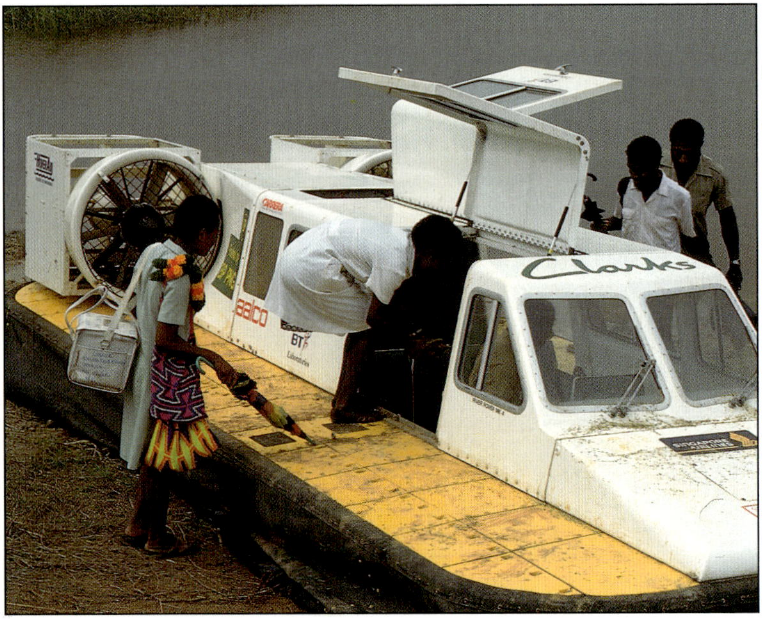

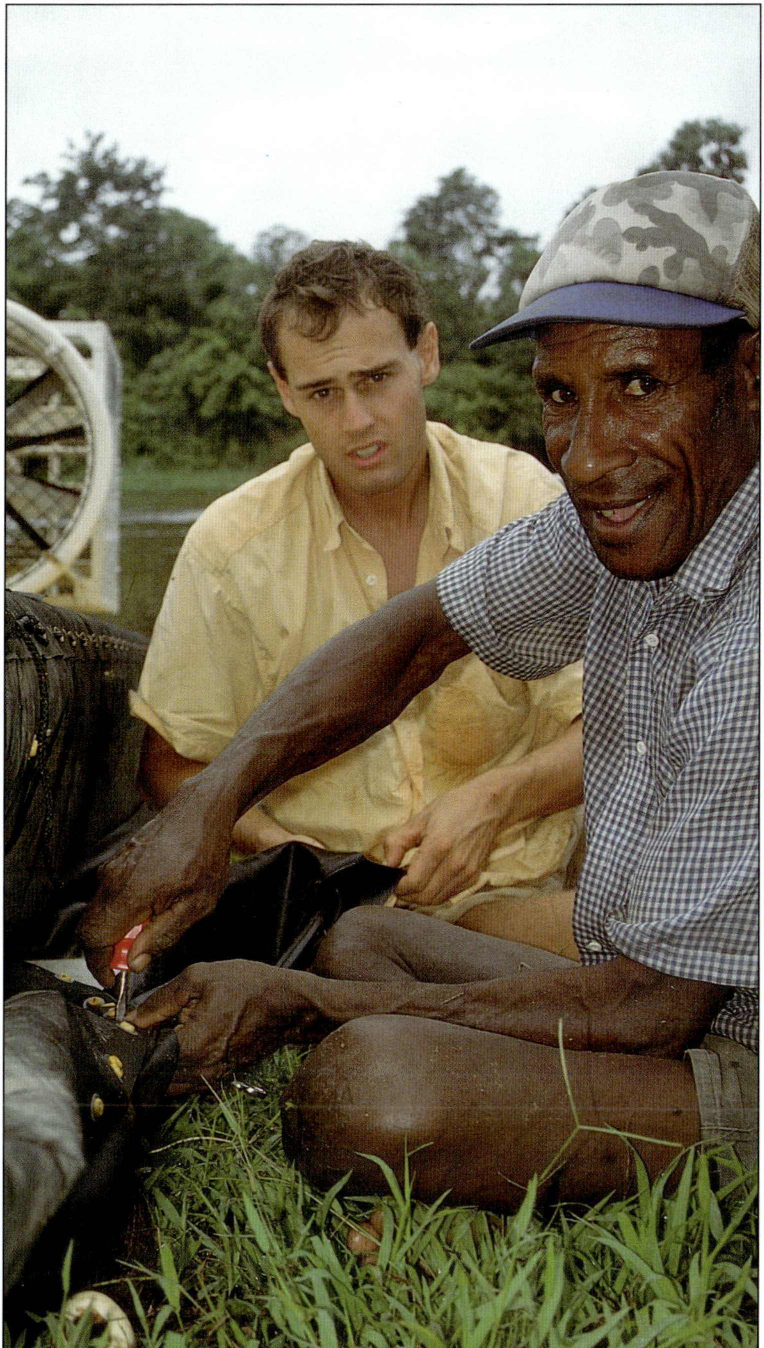

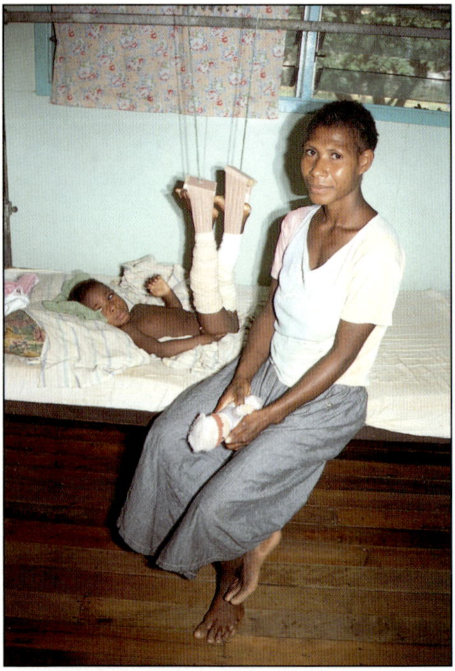

Left: Mother and baby at Balimo Hospital
Below: Village clinic with Graham Zerk
Right: Founding hoverdoctor Bill Gould and medical student Sarah Williams view progress on the garage
Below right: Parking for the night in the completed hover garage

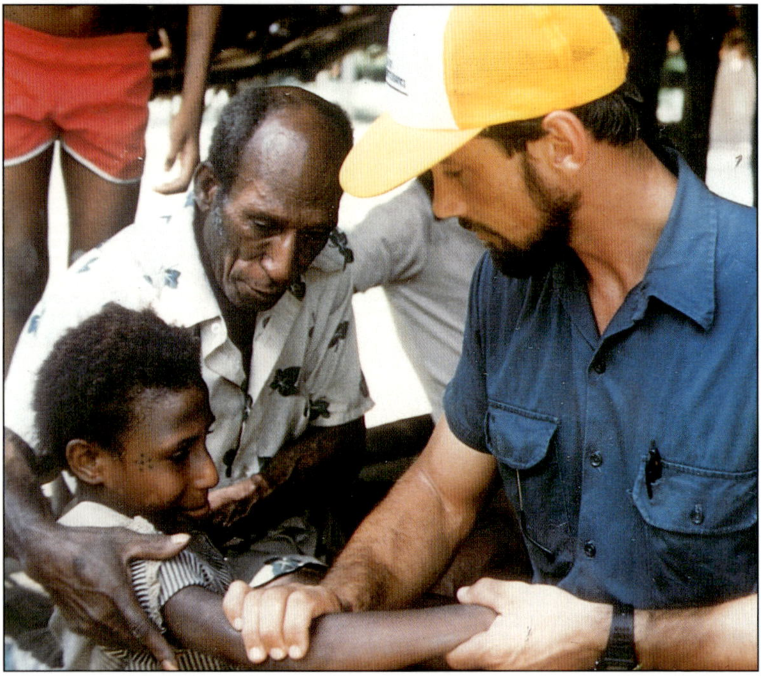

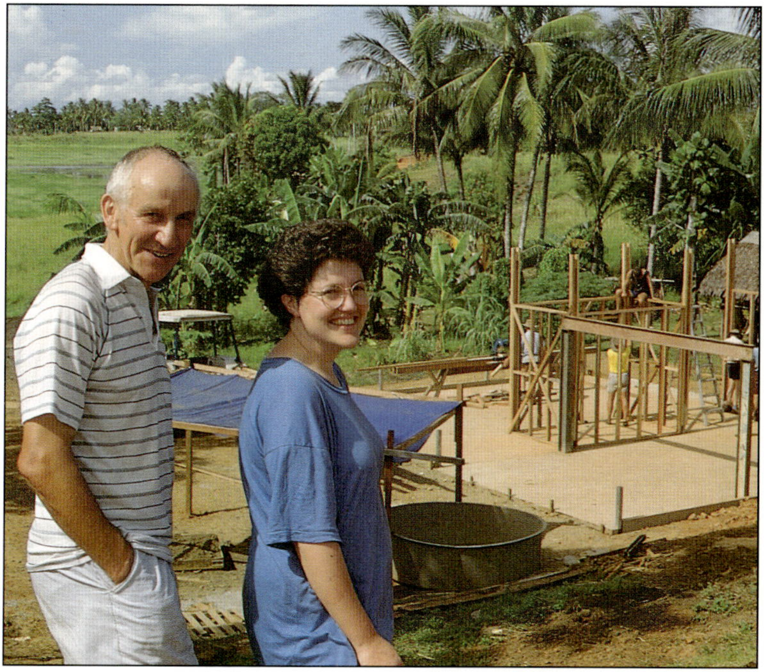

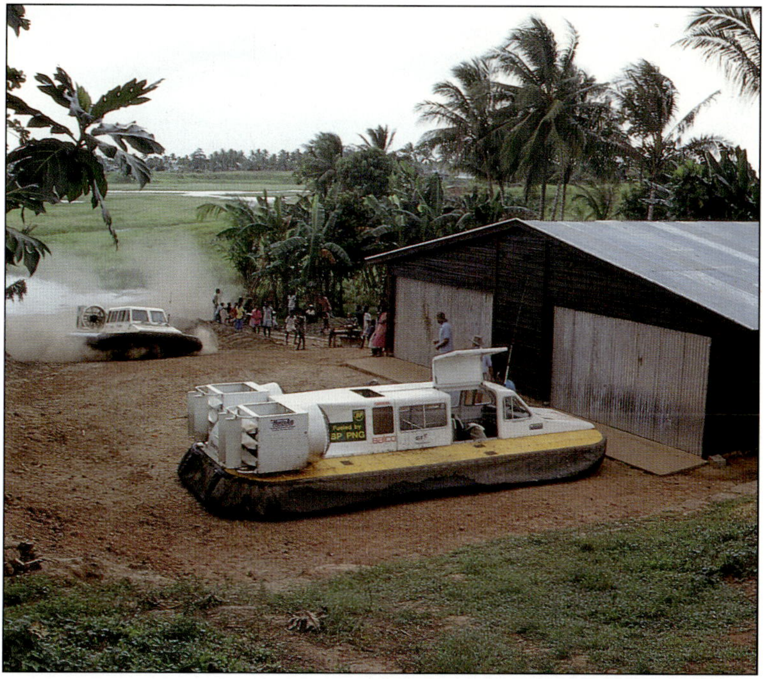
Fueled by
BP PNG

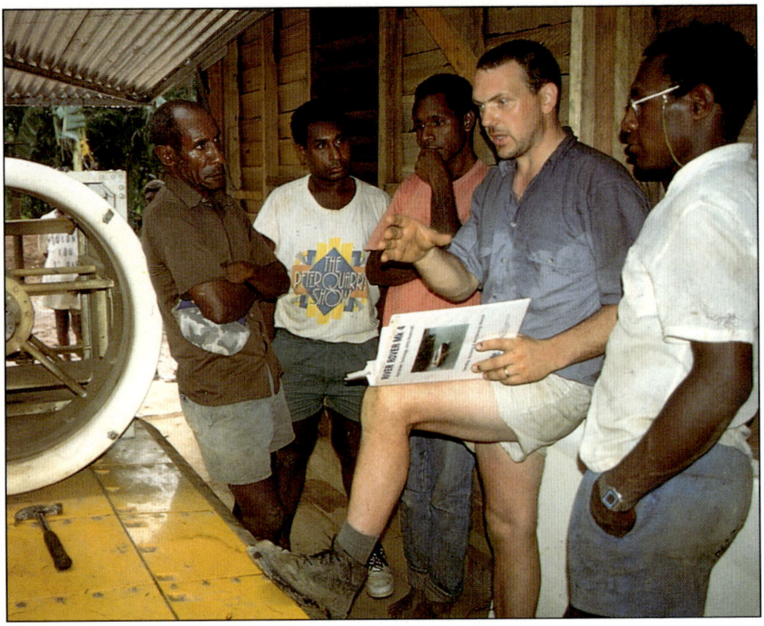

Above: Ground training for national hovercraft drivers
Below: Ola under instruction
Right: Sebia fixes hovercraft fingers

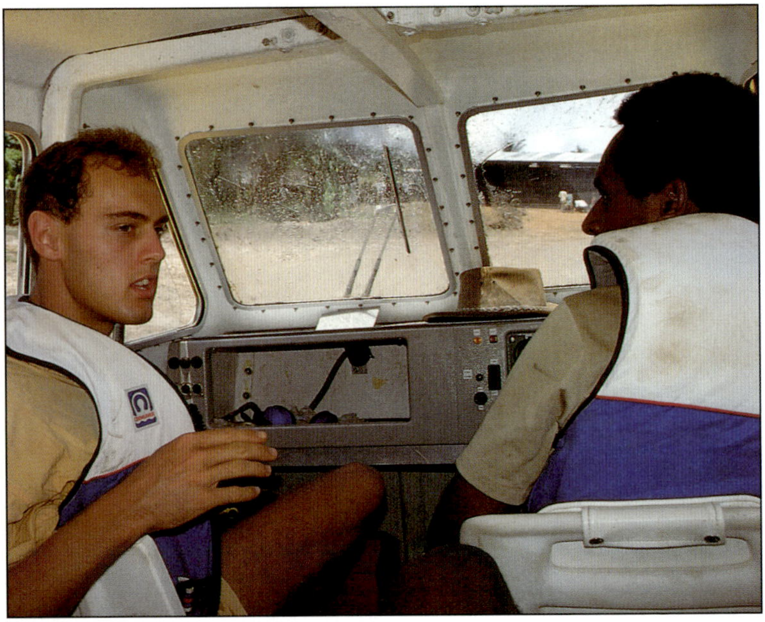

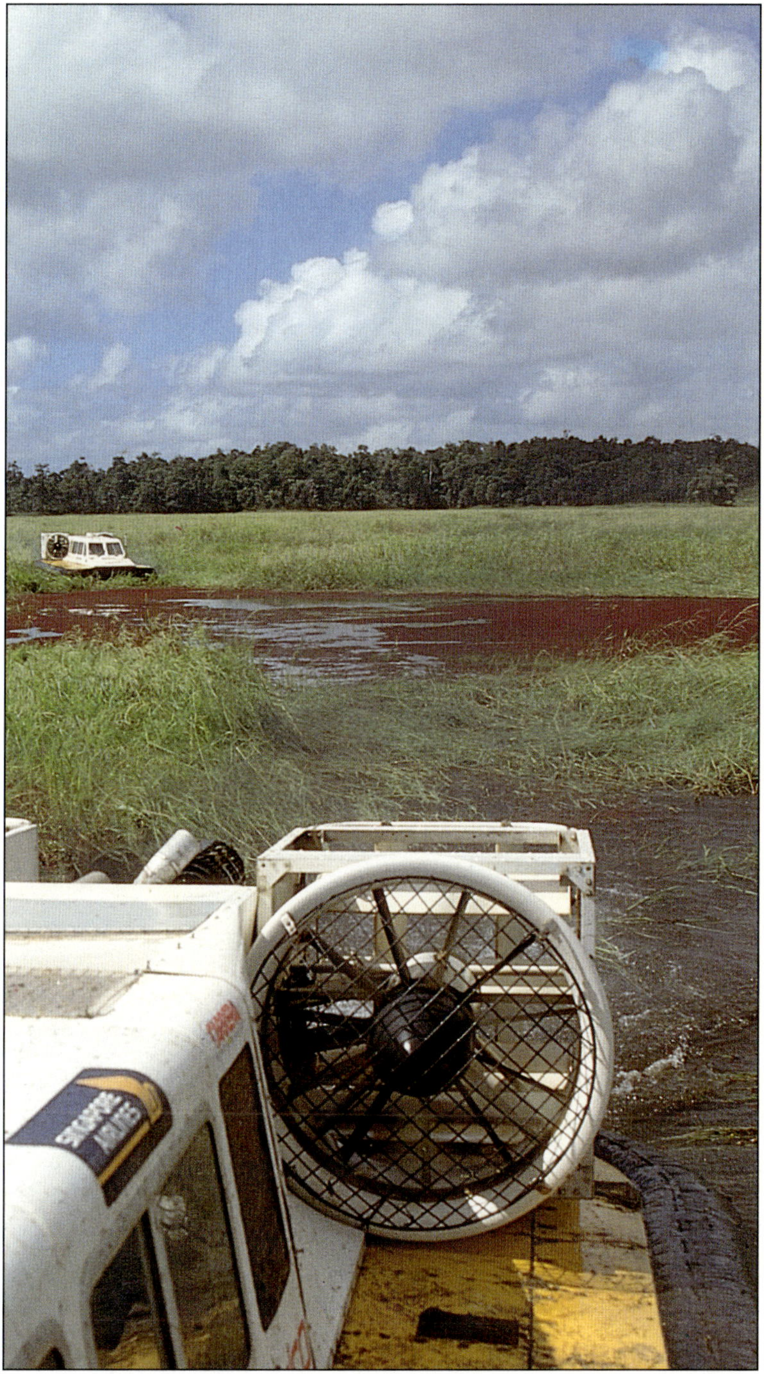

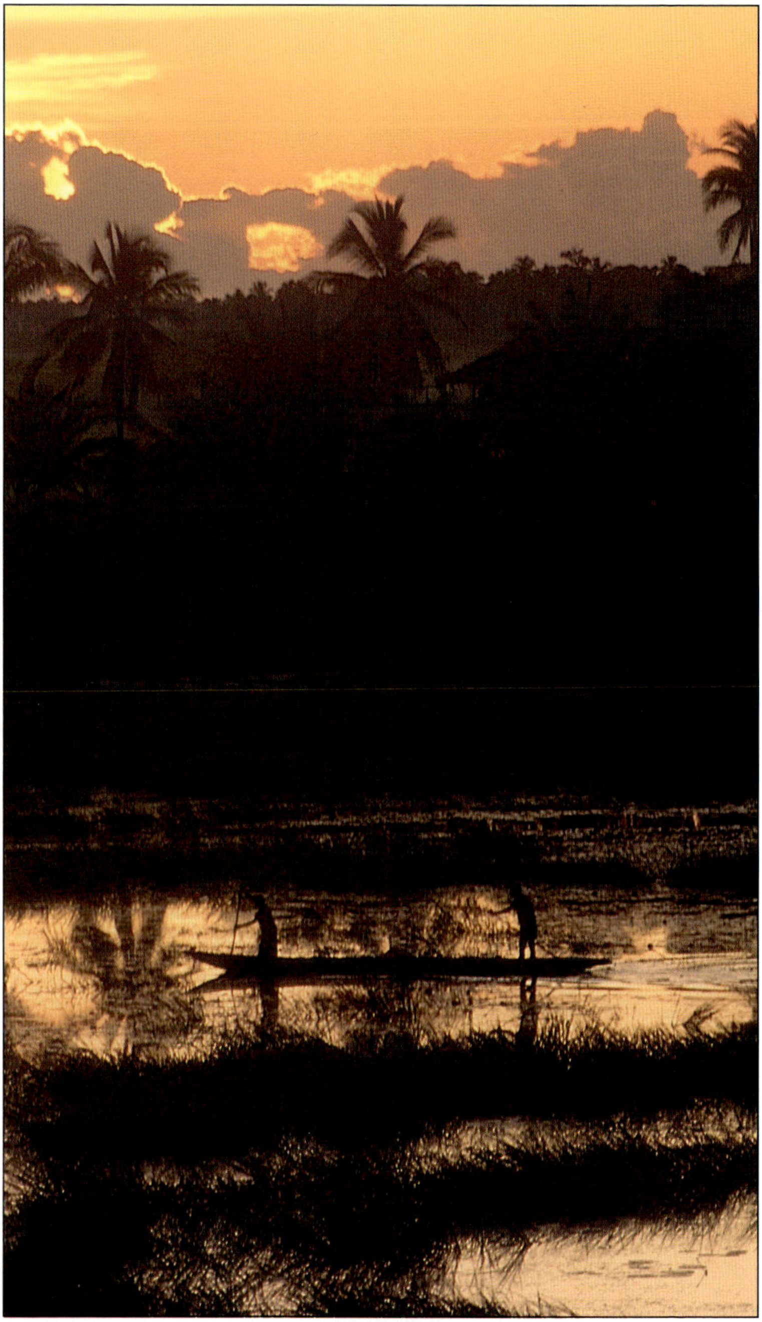

Sunrise over the lagoon

on its way. We asked the manager of the local shop to spread the news and started threading our way back through the mass of people. We need not have bothered about the crowd's reaction. These good-natured folk immediately headed off to the rugby match, clearly determined to make the most of the day and enjoy themselves, no matter what happened.

By the time we got back to our base there was further news and a major disappointment. River Rover was not going to arrive that day at all.

The turbo charger fitted to the Volkswagen six-cylinder diesel engine had failed. The craft had been unable to generate enough lift. The Volkswagen diesel had been specially selected because of its very good power-to-weight ratio. Reducing weight is vital because a hovercraft has to lift its own weight onto a cushion of pressurised air before it can make any forward progress. The failure of the turbo charger on a new engine was a major setback; it was totally unexpected, and we carried no spares. On the China expedition several spares had been carried, but they were never needed, despite the rugged and testing conditions. This engine was not a common one and getting parts quickly out to PNG, let alone to Balimo, might prove to be difficult. It was to avoid just that sort of problem for the future that we had to determine the list of spares that should be carried for operational purposes.

Anxious though we were to have details of what had happened, we tried to set those thoughts aside for a while. The hospital medical staff had planned a barbecue for us to celebrate the grand arrival. It had been a kind thought. River Rover had not arrived but the meat was defrosted and there was no point wasting it, so the barbecue was to go ahead. It looked as if our engineers were going to miss out, as they had not arrived back by the time we were due to start. Perhaps that was just as well; they in particular might not have enjoyed the empty irony of the intended celebration. Yet we could not turn down the wonderful hospitality of these gracious folk. We appreciated the opportunity to get to know some of them better, even though it could have been on a happier occasion.

It was a splendid meal and the setting was idyllic. We were sitting in the comparative cool of the evening, looking out over the lagoon, watching canoes slowly threading their way through the channels in the long water grass as the paddles dipped in unison and the blades glinted in the low evening sun. As the sun went down the sky was filled with glorious colour, bringing home with great emphasis the wonders of our God's creation. Soon, however, we were reminded of another aspect of it as the mossies started to bite and we had to clear away hurriedly.

Bill Ramsay and his wife Robin were there. Both are doctors who act as locums specialising in relieving hard-pressed missionary doctors in various places. Bill had come to relieve Graham Tucker so that he could take some leave and on his return have time to liaise with the hovercraft team.

Robin told me of a particular case Bill had dealt with. The Maupato family had brought their seven-year-old son Paul to the hospital recently. He had a large lump on his leg which concerned them. They lived in the Wawoi Falls area and had access to a health sub-centre, but the antibiotic treatment given there had not cured the problem. The Wawoi Falls are seventy-five miles (120 kilometres) away from the nearest hospital at Balimo and the family could not afford the air fare. The only alternative was a long and roundabout journey following the rivers and waterways. For three weeks the family had walked and travelled by canoe to bring Paul to the hospital. He had an abscess with a foreign body in it. Bill

Ramsay drained the abscess under a general anaesthetic and soon Paul was fit and able to return home.

At the beginning of the day in Kawito, Gareth and Ben had been on the job early, reinforced later by the arrival of more of the engineering team. By the time the launching party arrived, the remaining assembly tasks had been completed. The elevons and rudders had been adjusted, the craft refuelled and other final checks made. On their way up to Kawito the party had passed several large canoes heading downriver, packed with people. They were from villages along the river and were on their way to Balimo to see the triumphant arrival of the hovercraft.

The usual watching crowd of Gogodalas at Kawito had grown today to between 200 and 300. Whole families were out for the occasion, the young boys making the most of the opportunity to cool off by jumping in and out of the water in exuberant play. In imitation of traditional ceremonial practice, they had painted themselves with mud. Noticing Jonathan Allan's video camera at work they swung into an impromptu tribal dance on the river bank for his benefit, chanting in unison and prancing about stark naked.

Then came the big moment, starting up the machine. The engine had been run up quite successfully a couple of days earlier to check that all was well; there were no anxieties on that point. Now came the test of the assembly on which so many had worked. After a couple of coughs the engine fired and picked up. Clouds of fine red dust from the dry clay work site billowed into the air, smothering the team and the Gogodala helpers who had come forward to manoeuvre the craft into a launch position.

As the skirt filled, the hovercraft rose from the ground and started to slide down the slope towards the solid steel delivery container close by. A precautionary towrope attached to a tractor at the rear halted the craft in plenty of time. Heads down and eyes narrowed against the clouds of dust, the team and helpers pushed River Rover sideways away from the container so there would be a clear run down to the river. The rope was released and, gathering momentum, River Rover moved down the slope towards the water, only to collapse ignominiously into a spluttering heap a few yards away from the water's edge. In his excitement Dick had forgotten to open the fuel cock. The engine panels had to be raised and the fuel pump reprimed before they could try again.

The next attempt was more successful. As the skirt filled, Mike, who was driving, opened the elevons on the thrust fans and the craft moved forward in a swirl of dust to take to the water smoothly as the crowd cheered in excitement. The right elevons tilted upwards, reducing thrust on that side, and River Rover banked smartly to the right to move upriver, gathering speed amid increasing spray.

Impatiently the engineers on the bank waited for the spray to disappear, a sure sign that the craft had lifted over its own bow wave ('gone over hump'), so reducing resistance significantly. They waited and waited as River Rover laboured upriver, unable to get over hump. After an apparently successful launch, the craft was unable to develop enough power. It was just too much for Ben, who had laboured long and hard on the craft with Gareth. He let out an anguished shout: 'Oh, no! I just don't believe it!' He spoke for all the team members who were watching.

The crew of River Rover went through similar emotions: Dick kicked himself over the closed fuel cock and then, that problem solved, there was the excitement of that first exhilarating *swoosh* down onto the water; a surprisingly gentle transition from land to water. Turning right upriver Mike opened up the throttle, waiting for the 'kick in the pants' his twenty years' experience of hovercraft led him to expect. But there was no change. 'It just dribbled in,' he said later. Anticipating the disappearance of the spray as the craft gained power and climbed over 'hump', Dick urged the craft on.

'Come on, come on, what are you hanging about for? Get going, what's holding you back?' he said. And then to his great friend Mike, he added, 'Stop messing about, Cole, get on with it.'

'I am, Bell, shut up!' Mike said, almost twisting off the steering 'horns' in his efforts to push River Rover forward.

Then came the realisation that the craft wasn't going to make it, the disappointment, the puzzlement.

The crowds were waiting at Balimo. Very conscious of that, the crew racked their brains to come up with a solution which would get the craft there, even if with reduced performance. By now they had limped some distance upriver while they were trying to find an answer. Turning to head back to the launching point, they decided to try reducing the load. Mike put the craft alongside a small clear area on the bank and marooned Bill and Gordon there to be picked up later by Sea Rider. Pulling out into the river Mike and Dick anxiously waited to judge the effect. Mike opened up the elevons to maximum and gave the engine full revs. There was a marginal increase in speed.

'Give it more time, Mike,' said Dick encouragingly, 'it might pick up.'

'Okay, Dick, I'll try it,' said Mike, but without much conviction.

His doubts were well founded. As they went downriver past the launching point, the speed did increase a little, but still not enough to get over hump. They could not get to Balimo like this. Turning again, Mike headed back to their starting point. In a heavy mood he put the craft back on the bank in front of the now-silent and puzzled crowd.

At Balimo we anxiously awaited the return of the engineers, speculating on what had happened to cause the failure and what it would mean to our programme. As darkness fell and they had not returned, we were reminded of the difficulty of negotiating through the channels of the lagoon at night; no aiming points visible, the mosquitoes very active. Being stranded out there can be a very unnerving experience and once again, as earlier in the week, we could not avoid feeling rather helpless. We had no news of Mike and Co., except that they had left Kawito, and we had no way of making contact, as our only two hand-held VHF radios were on the boats.

It was not until long after dark that we received a telephone message via Graham Tucker to say the two boats had been sighted and the crews would need to be picked up. Tim went off with the tractor and trailer to collect them and their gear. He arrived at Hospital Point, expecting to see two tired and disappointed crews, but the place was totally devoid of any signs of life apart from the very obviously alive mosquitoes. It was dark and, apart from a faint reflected gleam on the water from the night sky, he could not see a thing.

After a considerable struggle and many false turns in the Sea Rider, Martin Healey, our own 'water rat', a skilled and experienced canoeist, had made it ashore somewhere, and managed to get a message through asking for transport before continuing towards Hospital Point. He then found great difficulty in picking out the right channel for the beaching point; every opening looked alike and there was not enough light to see more than a short distance ahead. Seeing a light on shore he assumed it was to guide him, but heading towards it he ran into a mass of water grasses as he missed a bend in the channel. Reversing, he went stern first into another patch of dense grass, clogging the propeller with weed.

Clearing a clogged propeller alone in the dark is a dispiriting experience, even though the outboard motor can be tilted to raise the propeller out of the water. Reaching out over the stern across water where crocodiles may lurk is not a task to be lightly undertaken with no help around, but Martin had no alternative as there was still no sign of the following hospital dinghy with the rest of the group aboard. Under power again, he could see two bright lights on shore. This time they really were for him — Tim had switched on the tractor headlights to guide him. But before he could get there, his petrol tank ran dry. By torchlight he transferred over to one of the reserve cans. Finally he made it into Hospital Point, where he was very glad to find Tim waiting for him.

Conscious of the time it had taken him to get in, Martin was concerned that there was still no sign of the dinghy. Knowing that the crew had far less water experience than himself, he decided to retrace his route to try to make contact and guide the other boat in. It was just as well he did so, for soon he spotted the dinghy making slow progress under paddle power alone. The extra load of the hovercraft crew had used up all the reserves of fuel. Martin passed over a spare can and after refuelling they were able to follow Sea Rider.

It was a tired, dirty and disappointed group who came out of the dark to rejoin the rest of us as we waited uneasily for news. We realised how they must be feeling and simply concentrated first on giving them food rather than pressing for details, despite our impatience. Relaxing over the meal, they brought us up to date before long; we in turn gave them our side of the story.

Many hours of discussion and speculation later, we had not come to terms with our disappointment. Maybe there was an element of injured pride for we had failed to deliver in front of those eager, expectant and admiring crowds. We had done all we possibly could, tried all we knew, brought the craft all the way from the UK. Yet we had failed to get River Rover from Kawito to Balimo that day. And we had a problem that had yet to be resolved. River Rover had performed well on trial in the UK, but not here. Could we put it all down to the turbocharger? Was it as simple as that, or was there a basic underlying problem of a machine that was underpowered? In the atmosphere of frustration and disappointment, earlier pessimistic doubts surfaced easily.

Gradually we realised that we had reached the end of anything we ourselves could achieve, and our only other resource was prayer. We had had another setback, on top of the days lost in Richmond. But we had our faith to fall back on, rather than sounding off in recrimination and bitterness.

Calmed and comforted by prayer we deferred any further action or discussion until later the next day, Sunday, and until after we had been to worship. There was time to stand back from the problem. The ten-hour time differential between PNG and the UK was in our favour. Monday morning our time would be long before offices opened for business that day in the UK. Fax messages and requests for spares could then be sent directly and quickly, taking advantage of the telephone line only recently connected to the hospital. It might even be possible to get spare parts sent out with Rachel Pinniger who, with our two medical students, would be leaving Heathrow late Wednesday evening.

So ended what should have been our big day. It was almost a week since we had arrived in Balimo. Much had been achieved despite our disappointment, and despite most of us having to cope with a demanding climate we were unaccustomed to. We had established our base; we had selected, cleared and levelled the site for the building we were to put up; we had assembled the hovercraft. But we had not got it up and running, and we had not got it to Balimo as we intended. Clearly the project was not going to hover without bother.

6

Finding Solutions

SUNRISE AT BALIMO is a truly amazing experience. Across the lagoon, beneath the stars of the night sky, the level line of treetops on the distant horizon is hardly visible. Faintly, as the sky lightens, a distinction emerges and then, as if a stagehand had thrown a lighting switch, mauves and pinks flow upwards from the horizon. Clouds, low above the treeline, appear in silhouette, rearing up as shapes in a fantasy, changing their form moment by moment as the colour floods higher, tinting the edge of the thinner grey clouds above. Reflected golden gleams appear on the open water of the lagoon, the grass between showing as dark patches of shadow as the shimmering pale gold creeps nearer and nearer. Palm fronds show in sharp relief against the lightening sky, revealing their delicacy and elegance. Suddenly, a harsher light spills like liquid in all directions, silhouetting fishing canoes against the water. Daylight has come.

This miraculous transformation from darkness to light, new every morning, shows the infinite variety and beauty of our God's creation. It gives us a new confidence at the start of our day and even the disappointments of the previous day are softened.

It seemed hardly possible that we had been there just a week; so much had happened. This was our first opportunity to attend a church service at Balimo. There were three churches in the area, all with Gogodala pastors; on the mission station and in the nearby village of Balimo the services are held in the Gogodala language, while beyond the hospital lies the English-Speaking Church, completed less than two years before with the help of Laurie and Andrew. It was attended by many of the hospital staff and we had been invited to join them on our first Sunday.

By 9 am the temperature was already well on its way towards the high eighties (about thirty degrees celsius) with a clear sky and brilliant sun, so we took the fifteen-minute walk at a measured pace. Unsure of where the church was, my small group fell in with some of the nursing school staff as they walked along the rutted dirt road. They led us to a simple, inconspicuous building opposite the rugby pitch. With our attention on the game we had not recognised it as a church the previous day. As we approached, the 'bell' started to sound, a length of steel pipe hanging from a chain, with a hefty steel bolt as a hammer. We could hear, too, the sound of singing and then some recitation in unison from the children's Sunday school being held before the main service.

Men entered up a flight of wooden steps to sit together on the left of the church; women went up an opposite flight and sat together on the right-hand side. Footwear was taken off and left on the steps outside. This was a matter of cleanliness rather than religious observance, for there was no seating and everyone sat Melanesian fashion, cross-legged on the polished hardwood floor. Most of us had not sat like that since our schooldays, and for some that was a long time ago. For support I sat against the open boarding of the side wall and benefited from the slight breeze it let in. The interior was plain but attractive. The rich timber of the roof beams complemented the floor; the pale decor and the shade from the deep overhang of the roof gave a cool appearance. A small, simple pulpit stood centrally on the edge of the platform at the front.

The congregation gathered quietly and patiently, waiting for the service to start. Pastor Lupiua started off the service with a greeting and then, on his guitar, led the singing of some songs. The singing was very harmonious and we knew some of the songs so we could join in. Later the pastor led a group of young people, accompanying them on his guitar, as they sang in pidgin English a song entitled 'Family bilong God':

Long marimari bilong God i salim Jisas i kam
Bungim yumi ananit long diwai klos

Yu no save long mi na mi no save long yu
Tasol nau Jisas i bungim yumi

Chorus

Yes, yes, yes, Yumi kum bun wantaim
Na kamap family, family, family bilong God

Not all the nursing staff were Gogodalas. Some came from tribes in other parts of PNG where pidgin was in general use; in the Fly area it is used little. During our attendances over the weeks, we were to hear many songs in pidgin reflecting the varied backgrounds of the nursing staff. The congregation grew in number as the service went on; more and more people kept arriving and gradually the earlier arrivals shuffled forwards on the floor to make more room. From time to time the service paused while people waiting outside were invited in and more shuffling created space for them. There was an informal open atmosphere in the meeting, in no way irreverent but with an ease suggesting that gathering together for worship was very much more part of the way of life here than it is in Western society.

Finally Dr Bill Ramsay gave a talk to the gathering and the service was rounded off with more singing. By this time, there was competition from the enthusiastic support being given to the rugby match which had started up on the adjoining pitch. We enjoyed the service, but it was a relief when it finished and we could stretch our limbs. Afterwards we had a pleasant time chatting to some of the congregation outside while our cramped muscles recovered. After the walk back, it was good to take up the Tuckers' offer and call in for tea and cake.

The different pace had been good, giving us time to relax after the bombardment of new experiences in the past two weeks; also to pause and take in the beauty of this area and appreciate its tranquillity, to adjust to its own tempo and rhythm. Some of us continued to relax in the afternoon, but not all; there were still yesterday's problems to address.

'Porridge-making' was Mike's irreverent description of the long meeting Gordon and the engineers had that afternoon. 'The more you put in to it the thicker it gets,' he claimed. It certainly had plenty of cooking time. The intention was twofold; to decide on action to cope with the turbocharger problem and to pool ideas and suggestions for improvements to the method of assembling of the craft. The latter would be useful when it came to the assembly of RR 402 in a few weeks' time. It might also identify suggestions that could be fed back to the HoverAid design and construction team. There was no shortage of ideas or comment and at times the temperature of the discussion rose as differences of view were vigorously contested.

As time wore on, I began to see what Mike was getting at. More and more points were being raised without conclusions being reached. It was becoming increasingly difficult to hold a clear idea of the ground that had been covered. Gradually issues were resolved and decisions made. Faxes were drafted to HoverAid, Volkswagen UK and to John Field's wife, Angela, who was acting as a contact point for us. She would alert Ray Pinniger that we might well need her to act as courier for some spares. The missing control cables for the Sea Rider had still not been found, so yet another fax was drafted to get replacements. The hospital fax machine would be working overtime the next morning. Finally a test programme was agreed to check on the reason for the hovercraft's lack of power and to experiment with temporary measures to overcome the problem with the turbocharger. That done, the rest could wait until tomorrow.

The rest of us relaxed that evening, but our two doctors had to be on duty. Earlier in the day an emergency surgery case had been flown in to the hospital. The patient's condition was beyond the capability of the hospital where she was being treated and she had been transferred to Balimo in a critical state. Before surgery could begin, the patient's condition had to be stabilised, so the operation could not be scheduled before 8.30 pm. Bill Gould and Rachel Grimmer from our team were to assist. The operation took one and a half hours and was not straightforward, as acute peritonitis was found. The patient's condition deteriorated during the operation but she improved afterwards and seemed to be set for recovery. Sadly, she died in the early hours of the morning. This was the third death in two days.

Monday's activities fell into three separate categories. The engineers had the problems of the hovercraft to address, they had to send off the various messages they had drafted for help and the delivery of spares, and they had to find a solution to the problem of getting River Rover to Balimo as soon as possible. The building work called for a small number to work on more site preparations before the labour-intensive work started and more of us could be brought in to help. Laurie, Andrew, Brian and John could cope with that work. That left the rest of the team available for some other activity.

Mike Cole was due to leave in a couple of days' time for South America, to deal with the work of the STEP teams there. He had planned to take the hovercraft up to Mapodo before he left. Helen Brackenbury, who was based there, had been involved in the first contact with Mike over the idea of using hovercraft in the Fly area. It was a pity Mike himself would not be able to show her the reality of the dream come true. Mike, Tim Goulding and I, had accumulated a number of letters and packages to take to Helen from friends at Gorsley, elsewhere in the UK, and from Balimo. We decided to go to Mapodo using more traditional transport, and a dugout canoe with an outboard motor was laid on. At the same time we could reconnoitre the route ready for the first hovercraft trip in that direction. As there was plenty of space in the canoe (or so we thought) we offered to take with us anyone else who could be spared.

Mapodo lies almost at the limit of the area that can be covered by the medical patrols until their range can be extended by using hovercraft. We travelled downriver in an easterly direction, that is, in the opposite direction from Kawito. It is possible only to refer to a general direction when travelling on these meandering rivers. The flat landscape is so extensive and the loops of the river so large that it is difficult to appreciate how much they do twist and turn around. The gentle sweep of the river takes the canoe so gradually around wide changes in direction that it is easy to become totally disorientated. I had a compass with me and the needle moved from side to side in a most bewildering fashion as the canoe went around bend after bend. Had it not been for checking on the position of the sun, one could easily have thought the compass was out of order.

Dick Bell was familiarising himself with one of the hand-held satellite navigation devices we had brought with us thanks to the sponsorship of British Telecom. The GPS (Global Positioning System) equipment would be valuable as we went further afield in the hovercraft. It constantly receives satellite signals that are translated into precise latitude and longitude co-ordinates, giving the position of the device to within a hundred yards (metres) anywhere in the world. Using that information against time, the GPS can also give a speed of travel. It showed that our dugout canoe was bowling downriver at a speed of almost fourteen knots.

With ten of us in the canoe the journey took two and a quarter hours, even with an outboard motor to push us along. We were sitting on a slatted wooden duckboard in the bottom of a narrow dugout canoe, our legs stretched out on either side of the person in front. Our bags were in front of us, between our legs. It was difficult to find a comfortable position and every change of posture had some effect on the passenger in front or behind. There was a limit to the number of permutations of position one could find. Extended legs went numb after a time; knees bent up suffered the same fate in turn. 'Pins and needles' followed each change. Taking one's weight on the forearm stretched along the rim of the canoe helped relieve the back for a while, but that too became very uncomfortable.

Eventually several of us adopted a cross-beam technique, sitting opposite each other and leaning against the side of the boat with legs diagonally across the canoe. There was a risk attached to getting into the position in the first place. The space was so narrow that it was necessary to lift your body up above the rim of the canoe to find room to turn. It felt precarious, and we had to move one at a time to avoid potentially disastrous results. It was best not to choose to carry out that manoeuvre when the no doubt expert helmsman powered the craft through a bend in the river and the canoe leaned at an alarming angle. All that apart, bowling along by canoe in the sunshine is without doubt a very pleasant way of viewing the riverside scenery.

Mike said as we piled into the canoe, 'All aboard the 101 for Paradise.' Mapodo is an idyllic spot, as he knew from his original visit. The approach from the river shows timber houses, high on their stilts, on a bank above the river and surrounded by coconut palms. In that respect Mapodo is similar to many of the settlements; it is only when one is standing on the higher land above the river can the true quality of the setting and the air of tranquillity it generates be appreciated. Originally built as a leprosy hospital, it was used for that purpose for only ten years before the government decided that treatment for leprosy should be given in general hospitals. It was then taken over by the Evangelical Church of Papua New Guinea (ECP) as a college for nationals wishing to serve their own communities as pastors or teachers. The original hospital design, almost ideal for that purpose, gave a spacious layout to the college. The combination of that layout, the backcloth of the jungle all around and the sweep of the river below justified Mike's comment. Immediately adjoining the college is a grass airstrip so MAF light planes can bring in supplies or fly out emergency cases from the Mapodo health sub-centre.

The students attend college on a four-weekly cycle. A very practical reason dictates that period; the sago they bring with them for their meals can be kept only for three weeks. After that it is no longer edible and must be replaced, so the students live at the college for three weeks, then return home for a week to gather in their sago supplies for the next period. This has the advantage of ensuring that they are not alienated from the way of life or diet of the communities to which they intend to return. The tribal culture of PNG, based as it is on small tribal groups, makes the nationals gregarious and very much dependent on the support of the group. To separate the students from that by using a Western-style educational term and giving a Western diet would cause assimilation difficulties when they returned to their tribe.

Helen, who had been at Mapodo for twenty-five years, introduced us to Wendy, who shares a house with her and works in the college office. These gracious and gentle women have considerable strength of character, an impression reinforced by a story Helen recounted. There is no electric light overnight as the power generator is switched off each evening at ten o'clock. Going to the bathroom by torchlight in the early hours of the morning, she realised that the unfamiliar black framing to the mirror was in fact a snake and, what was more, a poisonous one. Backing carefully out into the corridor she called to Wendy for help. Blearily, Wendy came and before she was awake enough to protest was given the job of keeping her torch on the snake to make sure it did not slide off into some unknown hiding spot while Helen went off to summon help.

Helen knew that the family of nationals in the next house had been having a family celebration late into the night and so thought that someone there would be awake to give help. Approaching, she saw that one of the elders was still sitting in his chair by the remains of a cooking fire in the area beneath the raised platform house. She called to him, not realising that he was dozing. Startled from his sleep, he stood up and turned around to face her, revealing in the light of her torch that he was stark naked! Modestly Helen turned her back while explaining her predicament and the old man, hurriedly dealing with his, stepped into his trousers with all the dignity he could muster. When they got back to her house she saw that he had picked up his hunting spear to deal with the snake but the spear was so long he could not manoeuvre it in the narrow corridor to get it into the bathroom. He calmly put down his spear, studied the snake and its position for a few moments in the torchlight and then with lightning speed pounced to grip the snake firmly behind the head before taking it outside to kill it.

We ate the sandwich lunch we had taken with us and topped it up with some delicious home-baked scones and cakes from Helen and Wendy. Surrounded by the tropical jungle our meal was, to put it mildly, incongruously English. Then we were taken to the college and introduced to some of the pupils. We met a group of young women in their late teens and early twenties who were the first female pupils to attend the college. They had already been out to two villages teaching Bible stories to the children by means of drama and pictures they had prepared themselves. Judging by their expressions the students were enjoying their time at the college. One had travelled from beyond the Fly River. Every four weeks she made the two-way journey crossing that wide and powerful river by canoe and then flying by MAF to Mapodo. These young people seem to count it a privilege to attend Bible school and are prepared to make a considerable effort to do so.

One class of young men at the college were mainly from the Tabo tribe, based further east down the Aramia River. The Tabo are mainly beyond the present reach and influence of the canoe-based medical patrols. The health standard of their villages is usually low, with no sanitation or clean water supply; as a result disease is rife, fertility low and life expectancy short. Some of the villages have no children below the age of five and slowly the communities are dying out. The same is true of many of the villages down the Bamu and into the Fly delta.

The young Tabo men were thrilled to have the opportunity of taking their education further, the first from their tribe to be able to do so. First they had to learn to speak Gogodala, for the lessons were given in that language. Until recently, their own language had no written form. Pride of place now among their books is a slim red-covered volume, Mark's Gospel translated into their own language. Tim Schlatter, a missionary linguist living with his wife and young family nearby at Saiwasi, had spent five years producing the translation. First he had to produce a written version of the language, and then he had to translate the scripture text into words and concepts they could understand; it is of limited value trying to translate Western cultural and linguistic concepts into a tribal language. They would be incomprehensible. It was a great pleasure to see the delight in the face of one of the Tabo young men and hear it in his voice as he proudly read aloud to us from Mark's Gospel in his own language, one of the few in his tribe who could do so. The ambition of these men is to go back to their villages to help pass on the benefits of their own education and to help improve the quality of life there.

Bill and Rachel could not resist going to see the Mapodo clinic while Dick and Mike inspected the airstrip, which to my inexperienced eye looked alarmingly short. By the time all that had been done, we were very much in need of a drink yet again. This time we were treated to water iced with cubes of frozen lemon juice from trees at Mapodo.

Finally we took a number of photos of Helen and the Gorsley trio standing up in the *Helen B*, a canoe adapted especially for Helen. It is two-thirds cut from a longer canoe and fitted to take an outboard motor. It has the reputation on the river of being a speedy craft and is well known as it carries Helen's own personal decorations painted for her in traditional style. Shortly before our visit Helen had been on a two-day trip when the propeller of the outboard motor was wrecked as it hit a submerged log, one of the common hazards of these rivers. Then, in two days, as Helen wrote to a friend, she spent 'fourteen hours paddling a canoe and got an unlooked-for suntan'. The outboard motor had reached the end of its useful life, and could not now be repaired, so leaving Helen without transport. Mike decided on the spot that at the end of the expedition we should pass on one of our outboard motors to Helen as a replacement. It would otherwise be sold to recoup part of our costs. We should have to trust that the money for it could be raised on our return.

We had quite a send-off as we boarded our canoe for home. The river bank was lined with waving children. We were saddened that we had not been able to show them the hovercraft on this occasion but promised to call in with it at some time as we travelled along the Aramia on our way to the Bamu River. The cross-beam technique proved its worth again on the journey home; it was made the more enjoyable as the passage of the canoe made the most of a pleasant breeze offsetting the strong afternoon sun. All in all, we agreed it had been a very enjoyable trip and we had many messages to carry back to Helen's friends and supporters at Gorsley.

In our absence there had been feverish activity by the engineering team. Making use of the hospital machine, the faxes drafted the day before had been sent far and wide. Not the people to sit around waiting for others to act, some of the engineers then went back to Kawito to see if anything else could be done to increase the power output of the hovercraft engine. They were keen to reduce the engine temperature which had been recorded at the extreme limit of the gauge at 239°F (115°C). In the high temperatures of PNG, it would be necessary to ensure a greater air flow through the radiator of the water-cooled engine. That could be achieved either by sealing off gaps in the engine compartment or by fitting an electrically operated radiator fan, as used on many cars. A plan was made to return the next day to make these modifications. Not having the hovercraft at Balimo was certainly wasting time; the sooner we could get River Rover to Balimo the better.

On the building site, further work had been done to achieve an absolutely level platform for the concrete floor slab. Drawing on his training as a civil engineer, John Field had taken over on the dumpy level aided by Brian holding the staff. Andrew had again been at work on the tractor with Laurie, both overseeing the site works and sorting timber for the structure. There were problems with the sawmill at Kawito and it might not be possible to obtain the length of timber we required for the main roof beams, which was causing Laurie some concern. We were coming up against more of the difficulties of working in this remote spot. With limited time to complete the work, we did not have the option of going further afield to look for other supplies; delivery would take far too long and we would have to improvise. It was becoming very clear that we were going to be a long way off putting up even the structural frame by Friday, when Laurie had to leave. As he had designed the building and drawn up the plans, Laurie was also concerned to pass on to us as much information as possible on the way he intended the structure to be put together so we could complete the building in his absence.

Brian's organisational mind had not switched off when his 'Bargemaster' duties finished; he had been worrying away at a problem while working on the site. How were we going to handle the heavy barrels of sand and gravel he had shipped over from Kawito? They each weighed one-third of a tonne. From his long practical experience he knew our untrained crew would be at risk of back injuries, crushed hands or feet. Getting the weighty barrels onto the site was no problem; Tim could handle that with the tractor. But we would need a way of moving them from the stock area without having to lift them. Then the sand and gravel had to be lifted up into the mixer with the cement and water.

Inspiration came as Brian ferreted around in the hospital workshop compound. Tucked away in a corner he found a heavy aluminium operating table, an old, discarded relic. To his fertile mind, this held the solution to part of the problem. Ingeniously he mounted it as a bench in front of the concrete mixer. Plastic buckets filled at ground level with the gravel mixture, cement and water in the right proportions could be lined up on the bench at just the right height for loading into the mixer drum avoiding the back-breaking job of shovelling the heavy material from ground level directly into the drum. A system of timber 'railway lines' was also devised along which the heavy barrels could be rolled after being dropped by the tractor, providing a very effective production line. Improvisation scored again! A heavy tarpaulin was suspended on posts over the operating table to provide essential shade for the mixing team. It also poured rainwater from the frequent torrential downpours into a large tank alongside the mixer, giving an immediate water supply.

All this work made for healthy appetites and someone had to feed the workers. John Field, our planning supremo, had calculated our needs and laid in stocks of items that could be stored. Catering for a team of twenty-plus people is demanding at the best of times. The complications of a restricted budget, limited choice and transportation problems only make the job even more onerous. There is no road access to Balimo from the rest of PNG, and the same is true with many of the settlements. All food supplies must come in on the Aramia River by ship, or by plane. The Mission Aviation Fellowship does not charge freight on food supplies flown in to the missionary stations, but food itself is expensive. The selection of food available is very limited, at least by the standards of pampered and affluent Westerners. Here all supplies of fresh fruit and vegetables must be flown in on a fortnightly schedule from the Highlands where they are grown. Vegetables do not keep well for two weeks in the PNG climate and there is inevitably wastage. Bread is brought in fortnightly but from Port Moresby, a two-hour flight away, and then frozen. Meat must be ordered in quantity directly from the slaughterhouse at Awaba, some distance upriver, and also stored in freezers.

Then there are the cooks; no corps of top-flight chefs these.

Some have no knowledge of cooking other than the smells that emerge from a kitchen. True, the labour force is leavened by a sprinkling of real talent, but coping with the novices will test the patience of the experts. The 'customers' also notice differences in standards from time to time.

So that the work should not fall too heavily on a small group, Gordon had asked John to draw up a rota of 'duty cooks'. Working in teams of four, the cooks were on duty for two days at a time with two new cooks coming on each day. The overlap gave a measure of continuity; leftovers from one day could be planned into the menu for the next day. While in theory the duty rota spread the work of cooking, it was not always easy to operate and ran into trouble when a cook's medical, engineering, building or other skills were required elsewhere. Necessary absences from base also interfered with the rota; medics might have to be away on hospital patrols. Generally there was a lot of give and take but occasionally there was some friction over the rota. Coping with these frustrations was yet another of the many lessons we all had to learn. Ordinary fruit was in short supply and expensive, but we needed a good supply of the 'fruits of the spirit' to cope with living and working together; they, too, can be costly!

7

The Healing Touch

IT WOULD BE SEVERAL days yet before we could finally get River Rover to Balimo and wipe out the frustration of the previous Saturday's failure. Meanwhile there was plenty to do, and the action helped us to feel more positive. The engineers were working on the hovercraft every day at Kawito and reports were encouraging. There was certainly plenty of work to be done on the building site. Rachel and Bill were spending time at the hospital helping on ward rounds and in the theatre, while still finding some time to get involved with our building work. We were always interested to hear what they had been doing and of the work about the hospital generally.

Our awareness of the hospital's work was growing in other ways, too. Our daily walk to the building site took us through the hospital buildings and the workshop at the rear and gradually we were getting to know some of the nursing and maintenance staff. Larry Mefaramu the hospital manager proved a great help, and we often had occasion to call in at his office on some matter or other. We were always made to feel welcome and his chilled water supply was a big attraction, too! It was good to develop our knowledge of the hospital's work. Increasingly we became aware of the great differences between the levels of health care available in PNG and in Britain, no matter what the deficiencies of the National Health Service.

The word 'hospital' does conjure up a certain stereotyped image, influenced perhaps by hospital dramas on television: the well-equipped ambulances delivering emergency cases on smooth-tyred stretchers; the staff whisking patients into spotlessly clean casualty departments, well equipped with supplies and specialised equipment; the experienced consultants available in every discipline. So much is expected and taken for granted in the Westernised world.

'Snakebite antidote was rushed 100 miles in a race to save a man bitten on both hands by his deadly rhinoceros viper,' began a brief report in a British national newspaper recently. The report explained that three separate police forces in Britain had linked up to rush serum from a privately run safari park to the hospital where the man was being treated. He was later described as 'stable, in intensive care'. The report was less than a dozen lines long and in the newspaper it was next to the much more prominent treatment given to a report on overcharging by a telephone company. The newspaper's priorities are revealing; it is relatively unremarkable in Britain to find public services combining in a medical emergency in a way that would be practically impossible in Papua. In the West we have more such advantages than we realise.

At Balimo Hospital the quality of treatment is excellent, but everything has to operate within very limited resources. I saw a notice about sticking plaster. A basic commodity in a hospital, surely? Prominently displayed, the notice set out the rationing system department by department, ward by ward, and stated the small number of rolls each could have. Supplies could not be guaranteed, it said, because of cost and uncertainty of delivery. And this in the referral hospital for the whole of the Western Province of PNG, serving 100,000 people.

The timber hospital buildings are of a high standard and equivalent to the best in the area. Like the local houses they are built on posts, although with floors raised not far above the ground. Inside, most places have painted partition walls and bare wooden floors. The decor is of the most basic kind. The windows of louvred glass are covered with fine wire gauze as a mosquito screen. Furnishings are practical: dated iron bedsteads, simple tables and cupboards, where there are any at all. Families camp around the beds of the patients, continuing to give close family support in sickness, often having travelled considerable distances to bring the patients for treatment. One ward reflects the patients' preferences even more directly by having no beds at all. Patients continue to sleep on the floor on the thin grass mats to which they are accustomed at home, their little bundles of possessions and provisions around them. Outside are the cooking huts where relatives can prepare food if they wish. The scene is far removed from the Westernised stereotype of a hospital.

The per capita expenditure on health care in the Western Province is about £3.50; in the UK it is almost one hundred times greater. A comparably sized general hospital in the so-called developed world would have at least ten consultants or specialists, each with his or her own junior medical or surgical staff. The Balimo Health Centre functions for most of the year with just two doctors who cope with all the general or specialist problems that come their way.

Yet this 120-bed hospital operated by the Evangelical Church of Papua New Guinea (ECP) is delivering a high-quality general hospital service that the people of the area would not receive if they were dependent on their government alone. The government gives an annual grant, unfortunately an inadequate one. The Minister for Health recognises that 'the churches have done the job better than the government'. The hospital has a modestly equipped theatre, supported by a laboratory providing a full range of services, an X-ray unit and a pharmacy. The range of wards covers the usual medical, surgical, orthopaedic, paediatric, obstetric and gynaecology wards. In addition there are wards specialising in malnutrition, tuberculosis and leprosy; an accident and emergency unit and a busy outpatient department which on average has more than a thousand attendances a week. Dental treatment is also available, and visits are made to schools. The Maternal Child Health (MCH) Clinic not only functions at Balimo, but operates village patrols. In the area covered most villages get a visit from a patrol each month.

Integrated with the hospital is a nursing school with fifty students. The annual intake is about fifteen students, of whom two or three are usually young men. A month of lectures is followed by two months' practical experience in the hospital and on medical patrols to local villages, then the cycle is repeated throughout the three-year course for qualification as a registered general nurse. The course prepares nurses to work in isolated rural settings. Diseases once rare in rural PNG are now included in the course: heart disease, alcoholism and diabetes. These are becoming increasingly prevalent, particularly in urban centres, and are thought to stem from changes in diet and living patterns.

Teaching is given in English. As that is a second language to most students misunderstandings can arise, according to Debbra Roberts, principal of the nursing school. One student, taught during a history lesson that Jesus Christ was born during the reign of Caesar, answered a test question by writing that 'Jesus was born during the rainy season'. Some letters in the language, such as 'p' and 'f', are interchangeable in PNG. Fat may serve pish for tea, for example, unless you're very careful.

Many qualifying nurses will go to serve in isolated rural communities where they will have to be able to diagnose and treat common medical problems with access to doctors only by two-way radio. This requires both the type of training given at Balimo and a willingness to go back and serve the communities they came from. Currently the government proposes to base all nurse training in the university at Moresby. The principle on which this proposal is based is being questioned, even in Western countries. In PNG it could result in a dearth of nurses willing to serve in the rural areas after training for three years in the capital, Port Moresby. The training needs to be to a high standard, but also it must address the practical day-to-day needs of the total community it is intended to serve. The Balimo school certainly does that.

Patrols going out to the villages are an important part of the work of the hospital. But nurses on a four-day patrol can spend a quarter of their time sitting in the bottom of a dugout canoe winding back and forth on the serpentine rivers and narrow creeks. By dramatically reducing the travel time spent on each patrol, the hovercraft will free much valuable skilled staff time and the villages can be given a more regular and more frequent patrol service. A rapid response ambulance service can also be provided using the hovercraft. Such a service can save lives.

But first we had to get RR 401 up and running effectively, get RR 402 into service too, and complete the hover-garage where the craft could be housed and maintained. We had barely started and many trials still lay ahead.

Trials and frustrations there certainly were for the engineers. While waiting for the replacement turbocharger, they had to puzzle out the reason for the very high operating temperature of the engine. It was exceptional, even allowing for the tropical climate and somehow it had to be reduced. Until a cause could be found and remedied, only the effect could be treated. One way was to fit a cooling fan on the radiator. Bruce Olsen was convinced that there was a suitable fan at Kawito but turning the workshop and stores upside down did not reveal it at first. Eventually the fan was found. Tim's skilful welding produced a bracket for it, and temperature control significantly improved. At last worthwhile trials could start on the river and performance worked up to a reasonable level even without the turbocharger to boost the power output.

Finally some progress was being made; not without a great deal of effort, for all the work had to be done two hours' travel away from base and out in the full sun. Being cramped for two hours in a narrow canoe, having to work with hot metal in dusty conditions, high temperatures and humidity and being in the canoe again for two hours before the relief of a shower and relaxation, does not necessarily get the best from the workers, nor does it produce the sweetest of tempers at the end of the day. Yet a sense of commitment was maintained and our end of the day get-together for fellowship and prayer eased any tensions..

Nor was Kawito the only place where the heat was on, in every sense. Rapid progress was needed on the building site before Laurie's time ran out and he had to return home. With that in mind, he was pushing on with preliminary work so that the next day many of the team could be set to work on the site. I was giving him a hand. Backwards and forwards we went across the site, with measuring tapes, string lines, nails and pieces of wood. To many an observer the process must have been mystifying. The whole business was to determine where holes should be dug to take the steel foundation posts. It was vital that the positions were accurate and that the walls were at right angles to each other. Tim used an attachment on the back of the tractor to bore holes into the ground to take the posts and the depth of the holes had to be exactly right. A makeshift scale was watched carefully as the oversized drill bored into the ground; frantic signs, accompanied by loud shouts over the noise of the tractor, stopped the operation at just the right level. Soil and lumps of clay spewed everywhere.

The carefully prepared site, initially cleaned off like a billiard table, was now covered with mounds of red clay, as though some huge mole had been at work. This was the sign for our 'barrow quartet' to strike up. Led energetically by Gordon on barrow, ably supported by Brian and Barbara on shovels, the mounds were removed one by one in strict tempo. Barbara, toughened by long years of hard work on her farm, shovelled away with the rest, setting a splendid example to those many years her junior. The finishing touches were provided by Martin H. Lying on the ground, arm half out of sight in the holes, he scooped out any reluctant lumps of clay, to leave a neat finish for the concrete bases. The red clay soil heavily stained our perspiration-soaked clothes, even if we did not throw ourselves on the ground like Martin. The damp, gritty paste quickly managed to get everywhere, leaving a red sandy residue in the shower tray at the end of every working day.

Everything was now ready for a major advance. Concreting could start the next day. A large team would be needed on site each day to handle the hard work of mixing the concrete; barrowing it across the site, compacting it in place and finally, with a light touch, smoothing it off. All this was to be done with only the most basic equipment and sheer hard labour: We must have been mad to do it in a tropical climate! Occasionally we staggered into the shade to pour water frantically down our throats and rest briefly to recover a little. Yet, in a way, we were loving every crazy minute of it.

By the end of the week the posts were in place and the low concrete base walls around the outside of the building had been cast. Almost to the last minute before his departure on the Friday, Laurie was into everything; directing the work, erecting wooden shuttering, organising timber deliveries, trying to cover a thousand and one details to ensure that all went well after he had left. His energy was amazing and he had clearly recovered from his 'Balimo tum'. Laurie held several master classes for Andrew, Gareth and me, talking us through the details of his design so we fully understood what needed to be done, and how. Andrew was to take over the lead organising role from Laurie, supported by the two of us. Thanks to Laurie's efforts the site was starting to take on some semblance of the hovercraft base it was intended to be.

On Saturday morning we had a sense of *déja vu*; River Rover was to arrive at Balimo that day. We fervently hoped it would make it this time; a second non-arrival was unthinkable. As before, the launch team went off to Kawito with Martin Healey driving Sea Rider and Jonathan in attendance, festooned with cameras to record the event for posterity. The arrival at Government Point was scheduled for one o'clock. That left many of us plenty of time to get in a worthwhile session on the building site where we descended in force. The routine was becoming familiar now. In no time at all, the mixer was in action and concrete was being poured in the first of the floor slabs. In typical style, and showing incredible energy despite the heat, Gareth was everywhere. Dashing around like a whirling dervish, he was directing, hurling buckets of gravel into the mixer, barrowing heavy loads of wet concrete across the site, opening barrels of gravel with hammer and chisel. Wherever there was anything to be done, he was there. Thanks to his energetic leadership and practical experience, great progress was made and instead of completing only one of the central slabs as intended, both were done, and by mid-morning at that.

As the last slab was finished Gareth, with great shouts of 'Yah hey!', leaped into the air several times, waving clenched fists above his head in an exuberant dance of triumph. This took us all by surprise and caused great merriment — a wonderful release of the tensions that had built up as we worked. Laughter is great therapy, and we certainly enjoyed a lot of it as we worked together. We came to anticipate Gareth's performances with pleasure as we neared various targets we had set ourselves. His antics were in no way contrived but were a natural expression of delight. This kind and gentle character, could drive himself with immense energy, and was a wonderful example to us all in many ways. It was typical of his open, strong character that, having lost an eye in an industrial accident some years before, he refused any artificial way of reducing the disfigurement. 'If I can live with it, I don't see why others shouldn't,' he insisted.

Almost as if on cue as the concreting finished, we had a visit from Pat Tucker. She appeared with a box under her arm. It was full of iced watermelon pieces, which to our parched mouths seemed like nectar. They were so cooling and refreshing. It was a very kind thought and oh! how we appreciated it.

As we neared Government Point the scene was a repeat of the previous Saturday. The crowds were just as large, if not larger; the previous week's failure had not deterred them. We were in good time for it was not yet one o'clock. As we went down the track we started to get cameras ready in case River Rover should arrive a little early, only to stand gaping in amazement at the scene that met us. There, sitting in its roped off enclosure on the water's edge, was River Rover. It had already arrived! We had not even heard its approach. Surrounding it was an excited and admiring crowd. Beyond in the water was Sea Rider.

The rest of the team were a bit miffed; everyone else had seen the arrival, but we had missed it. We had been looking forward eagerly to the moment of the first distant sighting: the hovercraft coming into view around the headland, the excitement of the crowd as they caught their first glimpse of the strange craft they had heard so much about, the speedy curving approach along the channel, the triumphant sweep up on to the shore. We had missed it and naturally we were disappointed.

The only thing we could now do was insist on an action replay for the photographs at least. This was an opportunity for Graham Tucker, Larry Mefaramu the hospital manager and Larry's young son to be given a first ride in the hovercraft. Many envious young boys saw them get in and go speeding off out of sight round the headland, only to reappear moments later and come sweeping up on to the shore in a flurry of noise and dust. It was still a thrilling moment, even though a little of the initial excitement had been lost.

Stage two of the arrival was to take River Rover to its permanent base for the first time. Dick, with Tim and myself on board as 'ballast', drove RR 401 out into the lagoon, feeling his way through the unfamiliar channels in the tall grass, not yet sure of the best route to take as he rounded the headland looking for a good way into Hospital Point. It was a wonderful scene as we powered in. There, on the slope above the site with the rest of the team, was a huge crowd, most of whom had hurried eagerly around from Government Point. The welcome was enthusiastic and as the hovercraft came to rest on the lower slope closer to the lagoon edge, the crowd came pouring down to get a closer look at this new machine, which was to become a familiar part of local life.

Crowding eagerly around, the Gogodala looked with questioning eyes at the craft. Close up, silent, and with the rubber skirt totally deflated, it looked lifeless. The hovercraft is a thing of movement, of water spray or clouds of dusts, of blasts of air; take those away and it looks strangely helpless, collapsed and rooted to the ground. Our task now was to ensure that the Gogodala themselves were able to harness the craft's unique qualities to the medical needs of their people.

The differences between the technological and the traditional Gogodala way of life were brought home to us the next day. John Field, Michael Pinkess and I were taken to Kini, a small village across the lagoon from Balimo. The journey to Kini took only half an hour in the dugout canoe using the outboard motor. Piliwa Kabawa and Duni Mulake had paddled for an hour when they came over from Kini to fetch us. They had no fuel for their outboard; fuel costs money and they had little enough of that. Thanks to the gift of premix fuel from Shell, we were able to provide fuel for the rest of their journeys that day.

Like all the villages of the area, Kini is set on higher land well above the water level, which was low for the time of year. The levels can vary, however, by as much as nine metres between the seasons. At times the villages can be separated from each other by huge inland seas. Cutting the motor, Duni skilfully guided us in through the narrow channel on the approach to the landing point. Other canoes of various sizes were drawn up on the shore, none with an outboard. Duni Mulake's skill is not limited to the canoe; he is secretary to the local group of carvers who are keeping alive some of the old traditional skills. He is also a deacon in the village church, of which Piliwa Kabawa is pastor. Waiting on the shore was a group of children of all ages; as we walked up the hill on the narrow track they followed in procession, some carrying our bags, which they were eager to take from us.

The sun, which until now had mercifully been tempered by broken cloud, lit up the scene in front of us as we topped the rise. On each side of the narrow ridge on which the track ran, huts were scattered at random, all set above ground on posts. As a backcloth to the hutted grassland were the ubiquitous coconut palms and some banana trees; beyond them was the jungle. The calf-height grass was heavily set with seeds which brushed off readily on socks and trousers, quickly working their way through the material on hooked barbs to irritate the skin. Wearing shorts and going bare-legged is the only practical answer.

Piliwa paid us the compliment of taking us to his home to meet his family, which gave us an opportunity to see one of the huts at close hand. Climbing up the widely spaced rungs of a roundwood open ladder, we felt privileged to be invited in and introduced to his wife, his sister and his five children. The house, we were told, had been built in one month with material collected from the nearby jungle. The custom is for the men of the village to work together as a group to build the homes for each other.

The scale of the house was modest — simply two rooms, one the general living room and the other the sleeping area. As guests we were honoured by being given straw mats to sit on, the rest of the family sitting directly on the split palm floor. There was no furniture. On one side of the main room was a recess with an earth hearth on which burned the cooking fire. A sago pancake was being cooked as we entered. A couple of rectangular shuttered openings in the walls served to give some light to the interior and to let out the smoke from the fire. The walls had a few texts and some election posters on them. The posters showed in black and white a typical biblical artist's illustration of the bearded Jesus and it carried the slogan 'Pray before you vote', which seemed sound advice. Some bowls, utensils and jugs completed the household equipment. The dim light of the interior complemented the scene. The house was cleanly swept and there was an atmosphere of quiet dignity about the family, who clearly took much pleasure from showing us their home.

Part of the reason for the simplicity of the setting became clearer when we learned that Pilawa, as pastor, earned only ten *kina* a month (about eight pounds sterling) on which to support his family. 'At times,' he confided rubbing the stubble on his chin, 'I cannot afford to buy razor blades.' How, then, did he manage to feed his family we enquired? 'Oh, we fish in the lagoon,' he said with a smile, pointing to a multi-pronged spear on the wall. 'We hunt wild pig and wallaby, gather coconuts and bananas, make sago; we get by.'

The Gogodala longhouse at Kini made an unusual setting for morning worship. It was in the course of renovation and large areas of sky showed through gaps in the roof covering; at the far end the roof was totally uncovered, exposing the timbers. The walls, too, were open all around and the jungle beyond could be seen through the framing of the building. Yet because of the sheer size of the whole structure, we were still conscious of being enclosed; we occupied only a small part of the floor area in the middle and the open floor stretched out a long way in every direction.

Few longhouses remain in the area now; each village used to have a longhouse as the communal home for the whole population, sometimes as many as 200 families living in the same building. Although built entirely of timber and other materials gathered from the surrounding jungle, the longhouses were on an imposing cathedral-like scale, the large central space extending like a nave from one end of the building to the other. This central chamber, the *komo*, was the exclusive domain of the men of the tribe, housing all the elaborate face masks and carved totems of the tribe and its clans. Spaced across the floor would be the earthen hearths around which the men would sometimes sit by day exchanging stories or legends and by which they would sleep at night. Enclosing the *komo*, two internal walls stretched from floor to sloping roof, forming side chambers. These were divided by floors to form upper stories in which the women and children lived, the boys graduating to join the men only after going through initiation ceremonies.

The main floor was reached from the ground below by sloping logs notched to form steps which could be pulled up when the village was under attack from warring neighbours. Beneath the building was a forest of stout poles set in the ground; some as supports for the main floor, others reaching upwards to carry the high roof. Sheltered by the sloping roof that extended down almost to ground level, this open area beneath the floor acted as a communal living space, dry and shaded, a place where firewood could be stored. Pigs — pets, food and part of the family wealth — were also housed here, and they benefited from the food scraps dropping through the gaps in the floor above. The longhouse was, in essence, the village itself. Today the villages consist of individual family dwellings.

The Kini longhouse had been built on strictly traditional lines as recently as the mid-1970s, to revive the fast-disappearing craft skills of the people and to act as a cultural centre. At the same time, a local carving co-operative was organised so that the traditions might be kept alive. The bowls of various designs, the model canoes with carved prows and the different fish and animal shapes produced are attractive examples of the carving skills of these quiet people. Unfortunately there is but a small local market for their goods. Without a life and purpose of its own and without a flow of tourists, the longhouse had been allowed to fall into disrepair. Now it is being restored and is currently in use as a church and general village meeting place. Even as we were leaving that morning, a call was going, out summoning people to a meeting to discuss some village matter. Symbolic of the contradictory lifestyles of PNG, where traditional dugouts often sport outboard motors, the call was being made on a battery-powered loud hailer.

People in PNG are relaxed about time and life in general, as seems the case in many tropical regions. Although we had arrived at Kini well before 10 am when the service was due to start, it was some time later when the 'bell' was sounded, calling the villagers to the service. As at Balimo, this simple but effective device was a section of steel pipe beaten with a spanner. It was surprisingly sonorous. Small groups of men, women and children were already scattered over part of the open floor as we went into the longhouse. People continued to arrive almost throughout the whole service. The informal atmosphere absorbed the movement of people, the wandering children, the noises of the babies, some being discreetly breastfed by their mothers, and the steady flow of new arrivals. Duni Mulake, for twenty-two years a radio and keyboard operator in the PNG Defence Force and now one of the church deacons, led the service and translated for us. He also led the singing, unaccompanied by instruments, unselfconsciously trying out several different notes before hitting one that satisfied him, and leading off.

The local Girls' Brigade started the service by singing an invitation to worship. They all wore simple shifts of royal blue with red sashes and their leader, possibly one of the grandmothers of the village, wore a red lanyard pinned to the shoulder of her grey dress as a badge of office. They sang harmoniously and vigorously, illustrating some of their songs with actions, stamping or running on the spot as they sang. Duni, sitting at a table immediately behind the girls, narrowly averted disaster by making a hasty grab at the two vases of flowers on the table as they toppled over to the vibrations of the springy floor.

Lunch had not been in our minds when we accepted the invitation to visit Kini. Our hosts had obviously thought otherwise. We were standing around after the service, chatting as best we could with our non-existent Gogodala and the villagers' limited English, when lunch started to appear. Several women carried in enamel dishes covered with cloths and placed them on a straw mat on the floor. The setting was completed with a couple of battered looking mugs and a plastic bottle of water, which had me fumbling surreptitiously for the Sterotabs I had put in my shirt pocket before leaving that morning.

At Pilawa's invitation we sat as best we could cross-legged on the floor and wondered what was in store for us. As the cloths were lifted to reveal dark green thick sausage-shaped parcels, we enquired politely what they might be. 'That's sago with coconut and pumpkin, and that's sago with pumpkin and fish, all wrapped and cooked in banana leaves.' I asked, 'Is the fish barramundi?' the only species I knew to be in the area.

'No, I was told, barramundi's not in season. This is another fish caught in the lagoon; it's very good but bony. Be careful!'

We three guests were handed enamel plates, the others made do with fingers only. Generously we were being invited to share what little they had, and there was nothing for it but to pitch in. Picking up the soggy warmish packets in our fingers and watching the others for a lead, we bit into the food. The unfamiliar texture and indeterminate taste were not easy for our Western palates to cope with, but we tried not to make that too obvious. Disposing of the fish bones proved not to be a problem, thanks to the split palm floor. The form was simply to drop the bony spines through the cracks.

John and Michael appeared to be coping much better than I was. Keen now for something to wash down the sticky sago, I anxiously eyed the water bottle and mugs. So far most of us had avoided major stomach upsets. Perhaps Pastor Pilawa sensed my thoughts for, rather diffidently, he enquired 'Do you have any water with you?' It seemed to come as a relief to him too as I hastily assured him, 'Yes, we brought our water bottles with us; is that all right?' Smiling, he nodded. Contaminated water is one of the most common sources of infection in the undeveloped areas of the world and we were both aware of that. We three pulled out our bottles and enjoyed the pure Balimo rainwater, grateful for the gracious way Pilawa had helped us over our dilemma.

Having managed to dispose of my sago *et al*, I was in for a surprise, much to the quiet amusement of John and Michael who must have sensed my reaction. I had put down my plate thinking I had finished when, to my concern, Duni started to pile on it several of the leaf-wrapped sago parcels. *Oh, no* I thought desperately, *I don't think I can cope with more.* To my relief he picked up the plate and gave it to one of the women to pass over to some deacons who were waiting patiently behind. Until then we had been the only ones eating, conscious of being under the scrutiny of most of the congregation, who were still sitting around. We had enjoyed being with these generous folk and had appreciated all they had done to welcome us. As Pilawa and Duni took us back to the canoe for the return journey to Balimo we were conscious, too, of the effort they had made to ferry us backwards and forwards.

We arrived back at Balimo in mid-afternoon and exchanged news on our activities. That morning Bill Gould had preached at the English-Speaking Church. By 4.30 pm he was Dr Bill again, operating on a little girl who had been brought in quite poorly — another possible case of peritonitis. From the tranquillity of the morning to the tension of a life-dependent operation; it was all in the normal run of things for Bill, but not for the rest of us.

8

Learning Curve

THE ENGINEERS WERE far from happy with RR 401, despite having got it to Balimo. There just was not enough power. No doubt the faulty turbocharger was the main reason, but they were bothered nevertheless. The replacement would be brought out by Ray Pinniger, but she would not be with us until the following week. In the meantime they tinkered whenever they could get their hands on the craft in between driver-training sessions, doing anything they could to increase the power output. Dick Bell was our experienced driver and it fell to him to train up a successor to take over his role when he returned to the UK in early April. Gordon selected Graeme Benke for the job; although an Australian, Graeme was also a serving RAF officer in the UK, who had been released from duties to take part in the expedition. As a young flying officer he was halfway through pilot training but such was the training backlog that he was unlikely to start the advanced part until well into 1994. Tall, tanned, and well proportioned with an engaging grin, he was always ready to take on any task, and he blended in well with the rest of the team. His quiet, patient manner was well suited to the role of instructor. Under Dick's tuition Graeme's first task would be training members of our own team; more importantly, he would then go on to select and train the nationals who would be responsible for operating the service after we returned home.

With Graeme as co-driver, Dick had first to develop the techniques needed to cope with the lagoon and the conditions that would be met in actual service beyond it, for that was where the greatest need lay. The conditions were very different from the rocky, turbulent Yangtze River rapids that Dick had experienced on the China expedition. The first requirement was learning how to deal with the grass. To go only where the coarse water grass permits would mean following the twisting channels the canoes have to use, significantly increasing journey time. It would be far better if the hovercraft could go straight through the grass. The ability to do this had potential benefit for patrols and ambulance work beyond the lagoon too. As water levels rise, vast areas of swampy land in the loops of the river are flooded. Then they become grassy swamp much like most of the lagoon at present. Testing River Rover's ability to overcome the grass was a high priority.

The open channels in the grass were best avoided by the hovercraft in order to reduce the risk for canoeists, which concerned the village elders. They were also bothered about possible damage to the many fishing nets fixed at the sides of existing channels. Discussions with them resulted in a decision to clear a wide, straight channel solely for the hovercraft as an approach route into Hospital Point. Initially the new channel would be cleared by the men of the village, working from their canoes and using long grass knives; thereafter the new route could be kept open by the craft themselves. Keeping to that line would avoid many of the local fishing and passage channels currently used. In future seasons conditions might be entirely different but as the craft would then be operated by local men, there should be no difficulty in sorting out a suitable method of working. Fishing nets were marked by long stakes showing well above the grass. Provided the stakes were avoided, there should be no risk to the nets; unlike an outboard motor the hovercraft did not have a propeller sticking down into the water to snag the nets and so could pass over the top of a submerged net without damaging it. Developing this understanding with the local community was important to the acceptance of the hovercraft as an asset; it must not be seen as a threat to their way of life.

Quickly Dick found that travelling at speeds over hump, when the hovercraft was going fast enough to mount its own bow wave, River Rover could plough long distances through the grass. If on taking a sharp bend the driver 'overcooked it', in Dick's words, the craft would take too wide a sweep and skid sideways into the grass on the outer edge of the bend. Then the chances were that the craft would drop below hump speed and have a struggle overcoming the resistance of the grass before regaining speed.

Reeds, however, were a quite different matter as Dick and Graeme found out — the hard way. Perhaps they were overconfident after the successes with the grass. The difference lay in the nature of the reed stems, and the fact that they grew on more solid ground or in shallow water. The coarse grass would press down into the water, leaving the surface for the hovercraft air cushion to bear on and form an adequate air seal around the skirt edges. The reeds' strong stems, by contrast, packed down on the ground below or in the shallow water to form a mat like a giant scouring pad beneath the skirt. The machine would then be stuck as the skirt edge failed to form a seal. Air pressure would be lost, leaving River Rover stranded like a beached whale. Once in this predicament, there was nothing for it but to get out and pull the coarse stems out from under the skirt until it could seal on the ground or water again.

It was an exhausting and filthy business. Often, once the craft was finally moving, it would stick again only a short distance further into the reed bed. Everything had to be repeated until the craft was clear of the reed bed, for there is no way of reversing out of a tricky position. A reversing system is under development for the River Rover series but is not yet available for field use.

Reeds also posed another threat. The lower edge of the hovercraft skirt is made up of flaps of tough rubberised material known as 'fingers'. These part around obstacles and then drop back into place to retain the essential air pressure on which the 'hover' depends. To minimise damage to the fingers they are joined to each other by sacrificial plastic bolts. These break under strain, so avoiding ripping of the fingers. The reeds were tough enough to snap a fair number of these links. On the first few encounters, not enough spares were being carried and so all the breaks could not be repaired. As a result, River Rover had to limp back to base under reduced lift, due to loss of air pressure.

These operational limitations had to be identified and overcome. Delays later could have life-threatening consequences when transferring a seriously ill patient to hospital.

It was extremely important for us to learn these lessons so that they could be passed on to the native drivers who were to be trained. Technological innovation, improvisation and problem-solving are not long-accustomed challenges in PNG. Used to the inherited knowledge of centuries of technological development, the Western mind can easily and arrogantly treat that knowledge as though it were an individual's personal achievement. It must be remembered that only just over sixty years ago, more than a million people were found living in small tribal groups in the previously undiscovered central highland valleys of PNG. They had never seen a man with a white skin and knew nothing about the use of the wheel. Within three years of that discovery aeroplanes were landing alongside their villages. Even the coastal areas have only been subject to the introduction of Western ideas and developments since the late nineteenth century. Such has been the pace of this nation's exposure to the technology that other races have taken centuries and even millennia to develop. But these are intelligent people, ready to learn at a fast pace given the opportunity and the means. The country has made staggering progress into nationhood since independence was granted in 1975, despite suffering many of the inevitable problems of an emerging nation. The developed world should give all the help it can, provided it can avoid passing on the failures of its own society.

Mike Cole had left us the previous week to go to South America and now Barbara Ferguson was about to leave. Barbara had raised some wonderful support from a group of churches in the Salisbury area of the Winchester diocese in England, enough to cover a significant part of the cost of the materials for the hover-garage as it had become known. Before she went, Gordon wanted to include her in a series of photographs for some of our commercial sponsors. We were all paraded in front of and on River Rover close to the lagoon edge, complete with various items of kit provided by sponsors: hats, shoes, sunglasses and sunhats, buoyancy aids, umbrellas, tee shirts and so on. Jenny repeatedly posed us to her satisfaction on River Rover as she instructed us which item was being featured in which shot. It really was a pantomime as we changed over from one product to another and it must have puzzled our usual Gogodala audience no end. But pantomime quickly changed to drama as we broke up from the last photograph. As we moved away from the side of the hovercraft where we had been posing, out from under the skirt slithered a Papuan black, one of the deadliest varieties of snake in PNG. Maybe we had disturbed the creature, but no one stayed around to speculate — it must have been the fastest photo call breakup on record! We had discovered that the Gogodalas are taught from the earliest age to deal with snakes first and ask questions about variety afterwards. On the shout of 'Snake!' they act very fast. Some ten- or twelve-year-old boys nearby grabbed long lengths of bamboo and in seconds had killed the snake before it had advanced more than a couple of metres towards them.

Spurred on by the excitement, Dick Bell then leapt forward with his all-purpose, all-singing and dancing giant Swiss Army knife and attempted to cut the head off the already dead snake — an unwise move, as we soon learned. For twenty minutes or so after death, these snakes are capable of inflicting a venomous bite by muscular contractions of the jaws. As the jaws close, the venom sac is compressed and the venom squeezed through the hollow fangs. If a finger or hand is caught in the contraction, the result is the same as being bitten by a live snake with potentially deadly results. Dick's guardian angel must have been at work, as he escaped this fate. In any case, his prized knife wasn't up to cutting tough snakeskin and the snake kept its head, even if Dick didn't.

As the driver training programme progressed, the range of the training runs extended, and before long Mapodo had the previously promised visit from River Rover. It took only one and a quarter hours, half the time of our journey by canoe a few weeks earlier. The advantages of the craft were clear, but weaknesses were also being discovered. One of the flexible hoses on the ill-fated turbocharger was found to have blown a hole. For the present only a temporary repair could be effected to enable the training to go on. By the end of that third week at Balimo it was time to start selecting the nationals for training. There were many applicants and it would be no easy task to select those with the right aptitudes and skills for this totally new role. Other tasks were also looming in the coming week.

After four weeks of living and working together, we had come to know each other fairly well. Individual characteristics, talents, strengths and weaknesses had been recognised and with all our differences we had become a team. Many adjustments had to be made for that to happen, and the process had not been without its tensions. Stable structures have the strength to contain these tensions; the less stable are torn apart by them. Although coming together as strangers, we had a tremendous advantage in our shared Christian faith — we all acknowledged the same Leader. That was the foundation of our team building but it was only the start. We still retained our own personalities and had to operate under the human leadership of one of the team with his own individual leadership style.

For Gordon Goodman the contrast was a considerable one. From the rigid authoritarian structure of the armed forces he now had to cope with a loose grouping of civilians of wide age range and widely varying skills, experience and responsibility levels. We must have been a difficult bunch, each with our own individual ideas and preferences. Put these in an unfamiliar environment, add an ambitious programme a limited budget, and the mix was a strong brew even for an energetic man of wide interests who loved being involved in the action. There must have been hardly a moment, apart from our times of prayer and fellowship, when Gordon could relax: there were constant problems to be solved, decisions to be taken, arrangements to be made and planning required. Every aspect of the work, every member of the team, was his responsibility, without the supportive structure and procedures of the service organisation to which he was accustomed. Not for him the comparative luxury of the more focused responsibilities of individual team members. Each of us in different ways felt our absence from home and loved ones, even though we had all freely chosen to be involved; and Gordon, an intensely loving family man, felt this too. All in all, it is not surprising that the quiet of the early morning found him alone with his Bible and in prayer, drawing strength for the day.

As breakfast finished, around 7.30 each morning, Gordon would stand up and summarise the events, achievements or problems of the previous day and then identify the programme for the day as he saw it. Inevitably there would be some factor or constraint he was unaware of that would have to be taken into account: 'But Gordon, before we can do that we have to ...', or, 'That'll have to wait. 401 needs to have its widgets tightened before Graeme can take it out' or 'No, the roof beams can't be finished today. We have to go up to the sawmill and ...' Possibly even worse was 'We can't have meat today, we've finished it, so it'll have to be noodles from the compo packs again.' There was always a reason why the plan put forward had to be adjusted at least in some aspect. Somehow Gordon managed to cope with all that and come up smiling, and a new plan for the day would emerge. Similarly on the job, with so many experts around, any suggested method was always open to question, or even set aside as new factors emerged while Gordon was away dealing with the next area of activity. These horses could be led to water but, ... ! Nevertheless, with a great deal of grace and goodwill somehow it worked, and things were done and done well. But it was demanding to have the responsibility of leading this disparate bunch.

Brian found that too, as the mantle fell on him for a time. There were other changes that week. Almost five weeks after we had left the UK, Bill Gould and John Field had to return home. Jonathan and Ben were off also, but in their case only as far as Port Moresby, where they were to supervise the offloading of the second hovercraft, River Rover 402, which was due to arrive there by ship at the end of the week. Once assembled it would be used in Port Moresby for a publicity launch before being shipped on to Balimo. Dick Bell was also going to help with the assembly of RR 402 for a few days on his way through Moresby as he, too, headed back to the UK. Gordon would travel to Moresby for the publicity event. On the way there he was going to visit his sister at Ukarumpa in the Highlands for two days and so he would be away for a full week. Brian was to be promoted to deputy leader for a brief time of glory.

At least that was how it seemed, but events made the role less attractive. It was not the work itself that caused the problem, for that was going well. Good progress was being made on the building; the selection of the national drivers was under way and the engineers had carried out servicing work on RR 401. No, it was that old problem of relationships that troubled the waters. To the young nurses training at Balimo, away from their home background for the first time and with little or no experience beyond that, the arrival of the hovercraft team and the future prospect of medical patrols in the new machines had a lot of glamour, as Brian was told by a nursing tutor. Add to that the presence on the team of eligible young men and the companionship of bright, warm young women experienced in travelling around the world, and there was a great attraction. This was fine and innocently enjoyed by all, especially at the joint Friday evening games of volley ball. However, it was proving to be a considerable distraction for the students and some of the senior nurses were concerned about that. There was also a rather a Victorian attitude to relationships between the sexes, so that the relative numbers of each sex permissible in any group became almost a matter of arithmetic. More care was needed.

The concern must have been building for some time, but it surfaced only when Brian took over. He appeared one evening looking distinctly shell-shocked after having been lectured on the subject by one of the nursing tutors. Then he had to broach the subject with our young people, who had only been acting in a friendly way, anxious not to give any appearance of prejudice or superiority. Earlier warnings had made them only too aware of the need not to offend local susceptibilities, and they had not thought they were dong anything of the sort. There was the matter of lights out time in the nurses' home; something we didn't know about. We all had an open invitation to join in the weekly evening fellowship meetings that the nurses organised. A number of us — not only the youngsters — had gone along, and had been made very welcome, perhaps too much so, for the chat afterwards had been very much enjoyed by everyone and had often only finished about a quarter to ten. This was not late by our standards but unknown to us lights out — literally as the power went off — was at ten and some of the nurses had been unable to shower before then, which was causing consternation. Unaware of this, our people would come home thinking all was well. Brian had his ear bent on the subject. The social tightrope was proving very easy to fall off occasionally.

Another of his trials was conflicting priorities. Fitting the various aspects of the work around the domestic schedules of the expedition was not always easy. Sometimes one of the duty cooks happened to be the person whose particular skills were essential elsewhere. Generally, it was left to the discretion of the cooks to decide on the relative priorities and how to cope with them. Many a time one of the duty cooks could be seen doing a different job elsewhere; it usually worked very well. But arrangements were sometimes strained, when someone wanted to be released to be involved with, for example, the nurses' fellowship. For Brian, struggling to be fair to everyone and to keep everything running on an even keel, such additional release was sometimes hard to accept. His point of view was not always understood by others who saw the much narrower picture of their own activities. Brian saw the absences as laying too great a burden on those left on duty and this led to friction on a few occasions, much to everyone's regret. Nevertheless, within the supportive atmosphere of the team, these matters were not just shrugged off as someone else's problem, but taken as part of the whole team's business. Because of that they healed up quickly. All in all, Brian was very ready to hand back command on Gordon's return.

Over in Port Moresby, Jonathan and Ben were once more enjoying the hospitality of the Olsen family. While installed in the transit house they were well looked after by Bruce and well fed by Kharen. That was just as well, for they had a lot to cope with. River Rover 402 had been shipped out from the UK by the Bank Line, one of our sponsors. It was, like RR 401, delivered in a steel container which was taken ashore at the wharf of Laurabada Shipping Services, agents for the Bank Line. Steve Holdsworth, Laurabada's general manager, was extremely helpful to us, and we owe him and Laurabada a great deal for all the help we received by way of storage and shipping services, not to mention the joy of taking refuge in his delightfully cool air-conditioned offices under the pretence of making a telephone call or sending off a fax.

Thanks to Steve Holdsworth, the container was placed in a Laurabada warehouse for unpacking. It was very hot in there, but at least it was out of the direct sun. With the help of Laurabada's skilful forklift truck drivers the stripped-down RR 402 was extracted from the container and placed on baulks of timber ready for reassembly. That left all the rest of the supplies, spares and tools in the container to be sorted out later. Gradually the workforce grew. Dick Bell arrived from Balimo on the Friday, Steve Moody from the UK on the Sunday, Gordon from Ukarumpa on Monday and later the same day I arrived from Balimo. The reassembly had to be done against the deadline of Thursday's launching ceremony. Invitations had been sent out to the press, representatives of our sponsors in PNG and various dignitaries. At Kawito the work had taken fifteen man-days; the schedule would be tight here, for everything had to be completed to allow for testing on the Wednesday. We could not risk any slip-up on the day of the ceremony. It was very reassuring to have Steve with us. His experience of the Mk III version of the craft on the China expedition as well as the building of the two diesel River Rovers, was invaluable. Though he was still jet-lagged and not yet acclimatised, his intense application to the job in hand was admirable. We were also well aware that he had left behind his wife with their four-week-old little girl; it was a great sacrifice by them both.

By 6.30 am on Tuesday the team was at work in the warehouse. We wanted to take advantage of the cooler part of the day and thought we needed the extra time, which we did, as we ran into some snags fitting the flow straightener blades in the fan housings. These were modifications fitted on RR 402 to give extra thrust. By late afternoon we were able to run up the engine for some tethered testing. Bruce, who had dropped us off earlier that morning, arrived back with his family, so we could give them a 'ride' in 402 as we did the tests. They were off to the Highlands the next day for the ECP Easter conference and so would miss the excitement of the actual launching. Bruce was staying until Good Friday to look after us and see us on our way back to Balimo before flying on to rejoin his family. The engine tests went well and we could plan to carry out a trial launch on the Wednesday morning.

But Murphy was giving us a reminder. His infamous law says: 'If anything can go wrong it will, and even if it can't, it might.' With the important ceremony the next day it was hard not to think of Murphy, particularly if he were to be proved right. We had manoeuvred RR 402 onto the wharf outside the shed. In a rehearsal for the next day, we were going to use the huge dockside crane to lift the craft across the dock basin to the slipway for a test launch and some runs in the harbour.

'I'll get those Phantom straps I brought. We can lift 402 with them,' Gordon said.

'Okay, thread them through the lifting eyes, then. I'll do this side, if you'll do the other,' said Steve, as he looped the immensely strong straps through the metal rings on the decking.

'Stand back,' Gordon shouted over the din of the crane engine. 'Lift away, up, up!' He waved to the crane driver.

The cab where the crane driver sat towered up above us, so

hand signals were the only means of communication. As Gordon waved to the driver, we stood back. That was just as well; the hovercraft had only just cleared the ground when ... *crack*! *crack*! Two of the lifting straps parted and River Rover crashed to the ground. Fortunately it had been lifted only a little way and the skids on the bottom of the hull took the force of the drop.

There was a moment's silence. Disaster had been narrowly avoided; a few seconds later and the craft would have been dangling high in the air when those straps parted as the crane swung sideways. 402 would have fallen with tremendous force on the sharp edge of the wharf. Five prayers of thanksgiving promptly winged their way upwards!

Sizing up the situation, the dockyard workers brought over some chains, which were then hooked onto the lifting eyes and looked much more secure. We stood back again and waved instructions to the crane driver. Nothing was happening; there was more frantic waving. 'Up, up!' we shouted, even though we couldn't be heard over the engine noise. Then we realised it was strangely quiet. The noise of the engine had stopped.

'Power's gone,' explained one of the dockside crew. 'It uses electricity. All the cranes do.' We hadn't given it a thought.

'It'll be off for at least an hour, maybe more,' said Bruce. 'We often have power cuts.'

'But we need to get River Rover onto the slipway so we can launch it. If we don't, we'll miss the tide,' said Gordon.

That was certainly true. It was not yet ten o'clock and already the tide was falling below the lower edge of the slipway ramp, exposing the concrete wall of the dock basin below. Another hour or so and the water would be far too low to launch the hovercraft and there was no longer slipway around. Without power for the crane, we were stuck; at least, it appeared so until Steve Moody, with his wide experience of the hovercraft, said, 'We can hover it around.' And so we could.

The narrow wharf in front of the Laurabada shed had access to the road, which served the dockside area. The yard where the slipway we had to reach was located also had a gate onto the road. Steve started up River Rover, sending the dust clouds flying from the dry concrete and the beaten earth. With many willing helpers from the dockside workforce, who had downed tools to watch what we were up to, Steve powered the craft forward into the main road. The rest of us were hanging onto ropes attached to help manoeuvre the craft on the narrow wharf. Unwisely, I chose one of the rear positions. Desperately trying to swing round the rear end as we headed into the road, I was dragged forward by my rope. The dust storm from the rear of the thrust fans completely enveloped me, blasting off my hat in the process. River Rover proved to be a real traffic-stopper, in every sense of the phrase. Huge lorries stopped for us, their drivers hanging out of their cabs to get a better view of the spectacle. Then with a wild swing our dust cloud made it through the gate near to the top of the slipway.

The tide had been falling while we had been overcoming the crane failure. By now the water level had dropped below the lip of the slipway. Steve decided River Rover could cope with the drop and, with Ben aboard as 'ballast' he drove the craft with gathering speed down the slope. Entering the water smoothly over the top of the wall, the craft found the drop no obstacle.

With the official ceremony now so near and with little time for adjustments, we almost held our breath as 402 went off down the basin. Would there be a repeat of the 401 problems? But there was not. Quickly climbing over hump the hovercraft, sparkling in the strong sunlight, raced out over the brilliant blue water of the harbour. After all the hard work, it was a wonderful sight. River Rover swept around the harbour at a brisk pace, tiny but dynamic against the anchored freighters and the hills beyond. Delighted at the performance, Steve did a number of test runs out into the harbour and said 'thank you' to some of our dockside helpers by taking them out as passengers before landing the craft.

The falling tide had uncovered more of the wall at the bottom of the slipway. Sliding down over the top when the water had been higher had been one thing. To Steve, heading rapidly back towards it at water level, the concrete wall looked high and hard. The crane was out of action, and we had no idea when it could be used to lift the craft out of the water again. There was little alternative. Steve took the decision. Opening the throttle, he headed straight for the wall. With a bang, the skids on the bottom of the hull took the impact as the craft mounted the top of the wall and staggered up the slope, seeming to expire with the effort as Steve cut the lift and the skirt collapsed. He had made it. All that remained now was to get the craft back into the shed and tidy away the area, ready for the ceremony next day.

The timing of the tide, which caused us a problem during the tests, was really a blessing for which we were very thankful. We had to fit in with the availability of the official guests when fixing the time of the launch ceremony and high-water time was the last thing we had been able to think of. It was not crucial, we had thought, as the crane could lower the hovercraft into the water. As matters were arranged for us, the starting time for the ceremony had been fixed at ten o'clock, precisely at high water on that day. It would be possible to have a dramatic launch of the craft down the slipway rather than an unimpressive dumping on the water by crane. Official guests could board directly from the dockside for trips out into the harbour. We had not been in control of the details ourselves, but everything had been co-ordinated for us.

The big day, like all the others we had had in Moresby, dawned bright and clear. Everything down at the wharf was ready so there was no need for us to be there very early. The Laurabada crew had done a splendid job in clearing up the area and by the time we had got the hovercraft in position and cleaned down, everything was ready well in advance. It was time for us to get cleaned up and ready for the ceremony to await the guests. Thanks to Steve Holdsworth and Laurabada Shipping, refreshments and cold drinks were laid on for after the ceremony. It was not long before the media arrived — a film crew from EM TV and a reporter from the Moresby *Courier*. Jonathan also had his camera set up to make our own video record and Bruce had brought along a small PA set that would be fully used later.

John Guy, the British High Commissioner to Papua New Guinea, was one of the first to arrive. Already he had been a great help to us and had backed official support with cash for materials we had to purchase in Port Moresby. It was good to have 'our man in PNG' fully behind us. He was soon joined by Bill Farmer, the Australian High Commissioner. One by one representatives of our PNG sponsors and well-wishers arrived and we were waiting only for the government representatives, Health Minister Francis Koimanrea and the Chairman of the National Council David Unagi.

With everyone present, John Guy started his speech, standing in front of River Rover. As he began, the steady low noise of traffic passing the wharf became a thunderous roar. The driver of a heavy haulage tractor unit, curious about what was going on, paused outside the wire mesh fence to lean out of his high cab to watch. The noise of his truck's engine reverberated from the opposite buildings and drowned what the High Commissioner was saying, despite the PA set he was using. Oblivious of the effect his truck was creating, the driver waited until John Guy had finished and then, curiosity satisfied, drove off. Gordon was able to reply to the High Commissioner's speech without noisy competition and then the Health Minister gave his welcome.

With the Health Minister, High Commissioner and Chairman of the National Council aboard, Gordon drove RR 402 out for the official inaugural run. The tide level was perfect, just lapping onto the lip of the slipway and giving a smooth transition from concrete to water. As River Rover sped away down the loading basin and out into the harbour, we could not have wished for more. The TV camera was recording the event, as was Jonathan's, and the newspaper reporter was scribbling furiously. The launch was certainly getting good press attention. On his return, Francis Koimanrea made a very encouraging speech, suggesting that other places in PNG could benefit from this technology.

Steve Moody took over the driving next, and gave our sponsors' representatives and the media an opportunity of experiencing the craft for themselves, while the rest went into the shade of the warehouse for refreshments. Gordon was whisked off for a radio chat show and Jonathan took advantage of the keen TV interest to go off to the studios with the film crew. He needed to copy some videotape to send back to the UK for Bill Gould to add to a BBC news item about the medical work.

All in all, it had been an enjoyable morning. We celebrated by lunching out with Bruce, Ron Smith and his helpers, all of whom had worked hard to make the occasion successful. Later we relaxed further by taking a dip in a Moresby open-air swimming pool in unheated water that had the temperature of a warm bath. In the evening we watched the TV news item and thought it gave a fair report.

The next stage was to get the second hovercraft to Balimo. Jonathan stayed behind in Moresby to supervise the loading of the craft onto the ship that would take it. A number of spares were also needed there without delay and we wanted him to ensure they, too, were loaded. The next day, Steve, Gordon, Ben and I packed up and headed for the airport, keen to get back into action.

9

On Patrol and Up the Creek

THE RAIN WAS SLUICING down as the medical patrol left Balimo. It would take five hours to get to Wasapea where the first clinic would be held, and the dugout canoe offered the patrol no protection. Despite the canvas sheet draped over their, kit most of it was wet when they stopped at Awaba for a break almost three hours later. Dr Ray Pinniger and Sarah Williams, one of our two medical students, were off on one of the regular four-day patrols, heading westwards along the Aramia from Balimo. Six nurses, one male, and a boatman made up the rest of the Maternal Child Health (MCH) patrol.

The patrol would be on the move for five days, calling at five villages strung out along the river; almost 200 hours of skilled medical time would be lost in travelling by canoe. Wasapea and Makapa have no medical services at all; Kaniya and Ali each have a simple aid post, staffed by an orderly. Only Awaba, where they would first break their journey, has a health sub-centre staffed by four nursing sisters. Anyone at Ali needing hospital attention has to face a minimum six-hour journey in an outboard powered open canoe to the nearest airstrip at Awaba, if they can afford the cost of a flight to Balimo; otherwise, the journey takes up to twenty hours, paddling all the way. Whatever the mode of transport, it's a long time before the sick person can see a doctor.

With a brief break at Awaba, there was just time to hold a clinic at Wasapea and then reach Kaniya before dark. As they approached Wasapea, they were greeted by the typical village scene of sago-thatched huts on stilts. Heading for the church, they prepared to hold a clinic. Villagers were summoned by simply ringing the church 'bell'. Mothers came clutching record cards, to have their babies weighed and measured and their sores treated. The weighing and measuring is a good first assessment of child development which can indicate any lack of normal growth due to malnutrition. Immunisations can be carried out at the same time. The attendance was not as good as usual, since many of the families had been away to an event at Awaba and had not yet returned. Until the establishment of a regular programme of visits on the same day each month, it will be difficult to maintain any continuity of monitoring.

As the light was failing they approached Kaniya, turning up a narrow creek off the main river. The boatman cut the engine as the water shallowed and out came the paddles. As the canoe ran aground, Sarah jumped out to lighten the load — right up to her knees in mud and water. With a few heaves they made it in to the landing point. Waiting for them were the village children, who hooted with laughter at the sight of Sarah's muddy, dripping wet Ali Baba trousers as she squelched ashore. Sarah has a wonderful ability to communicate with children through the simplest of actions or expressions.

There was no shortage of volunteer porters to carry their equipment and personal kit up to the church where they were to

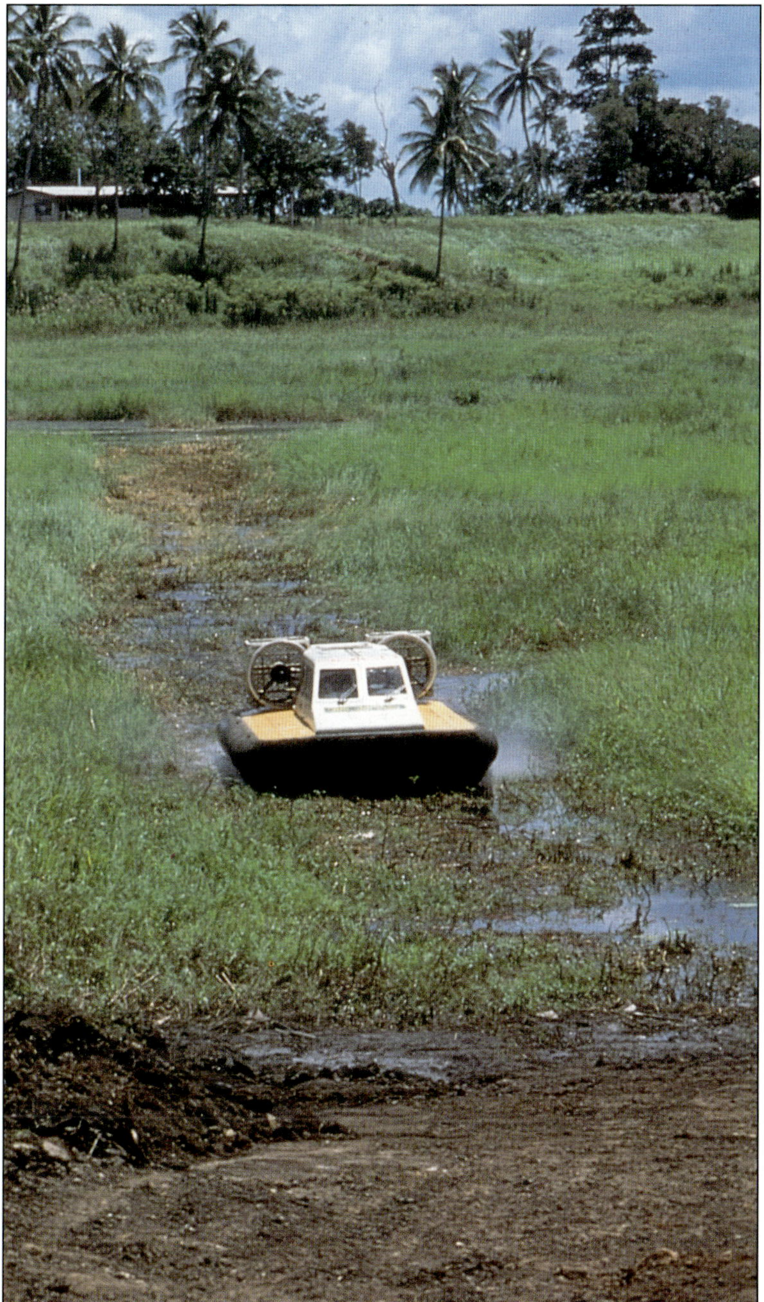

Across the lagoon

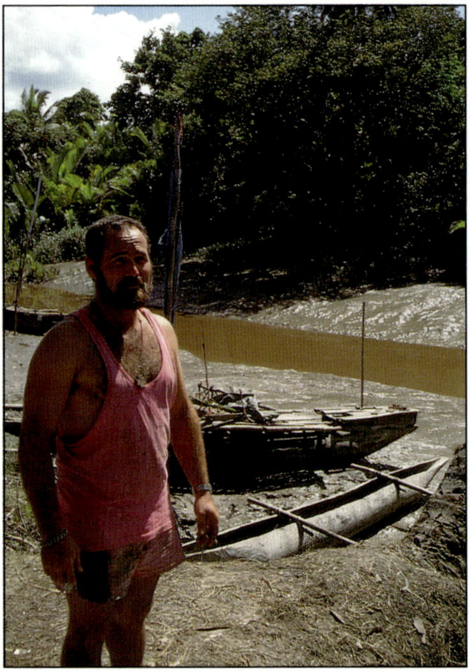

Left: Father Ron at Sisiama
Below: Sisiama village
Right: Pass on the left
Below right: Overnight protection from the mosquito

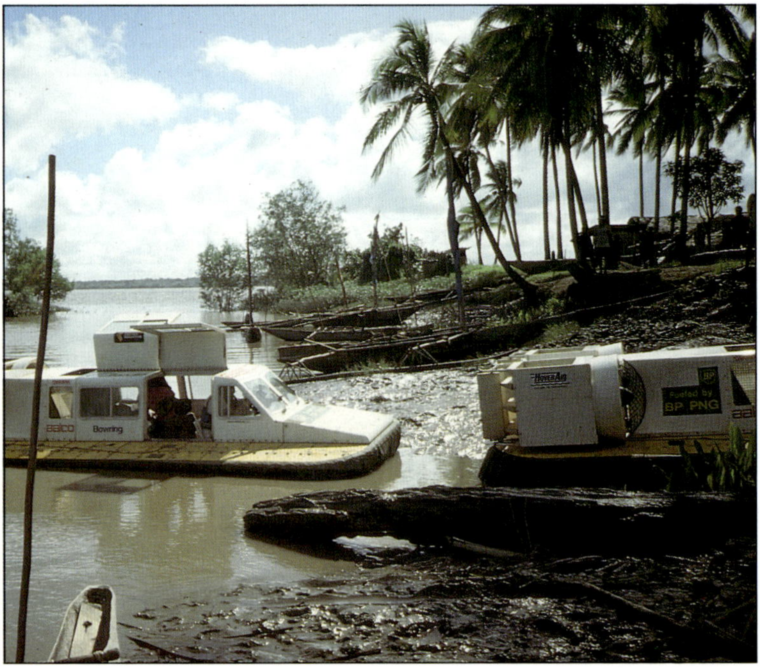

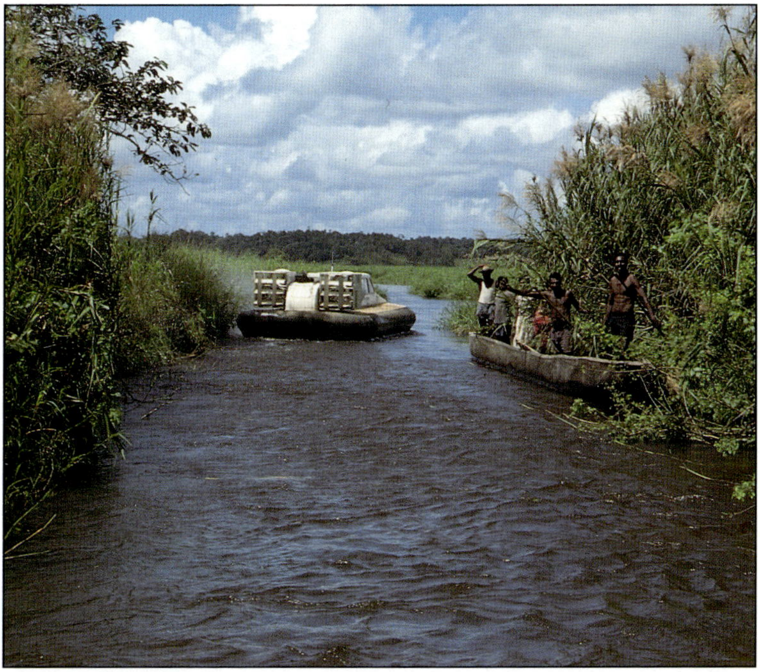

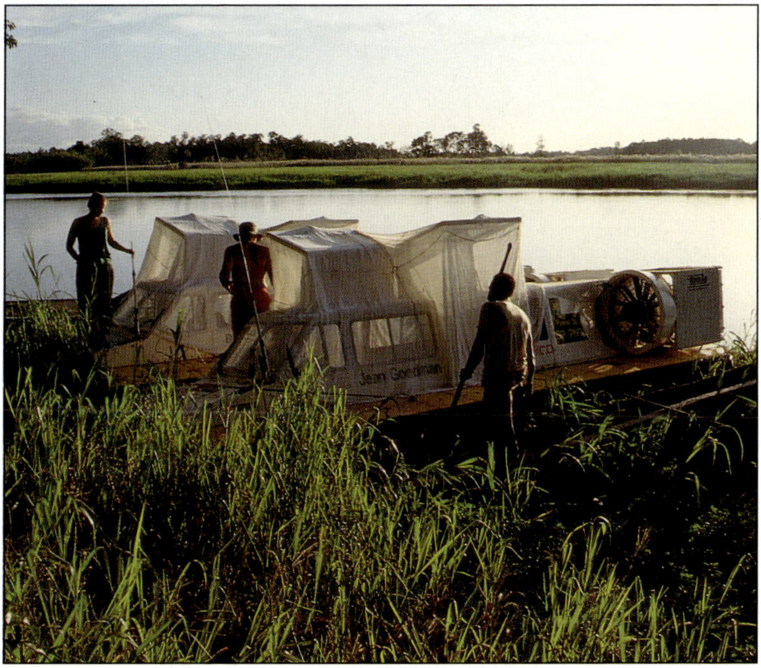

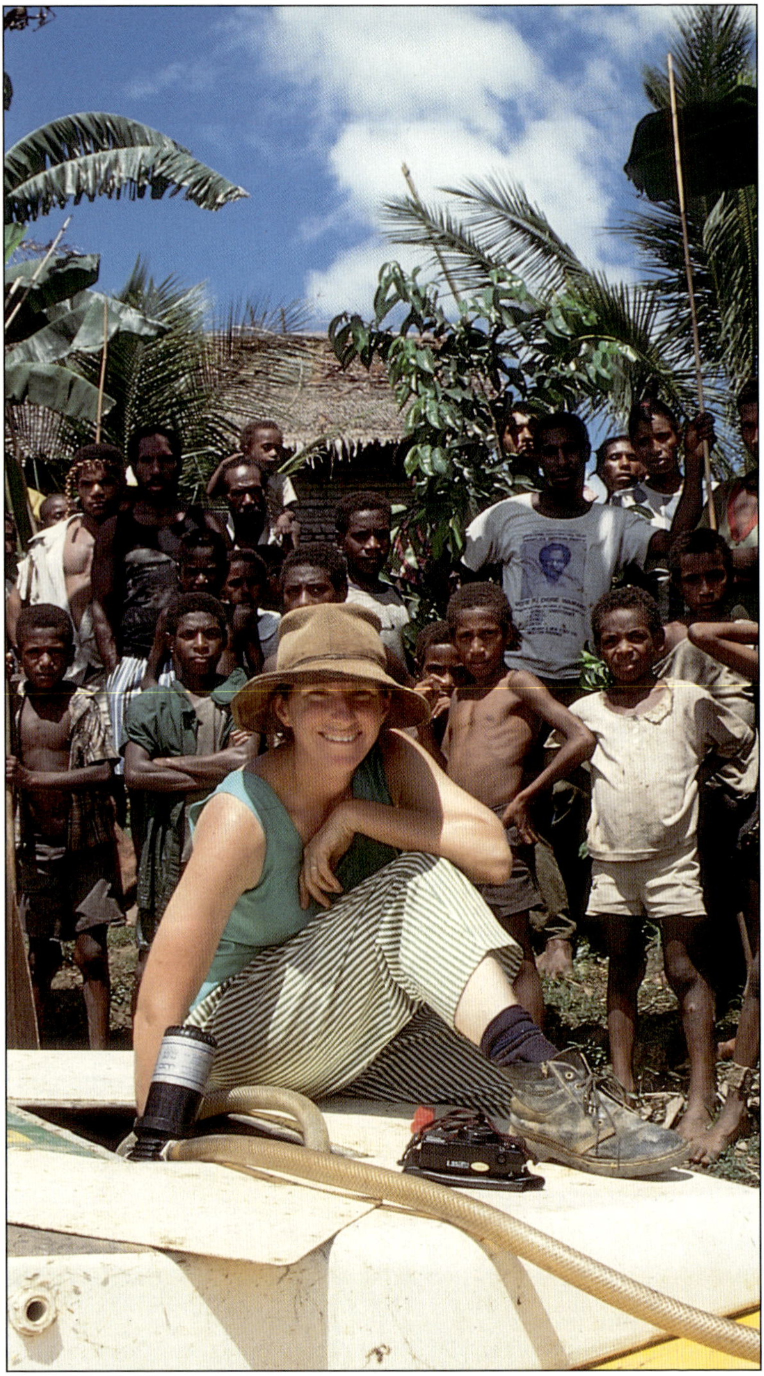

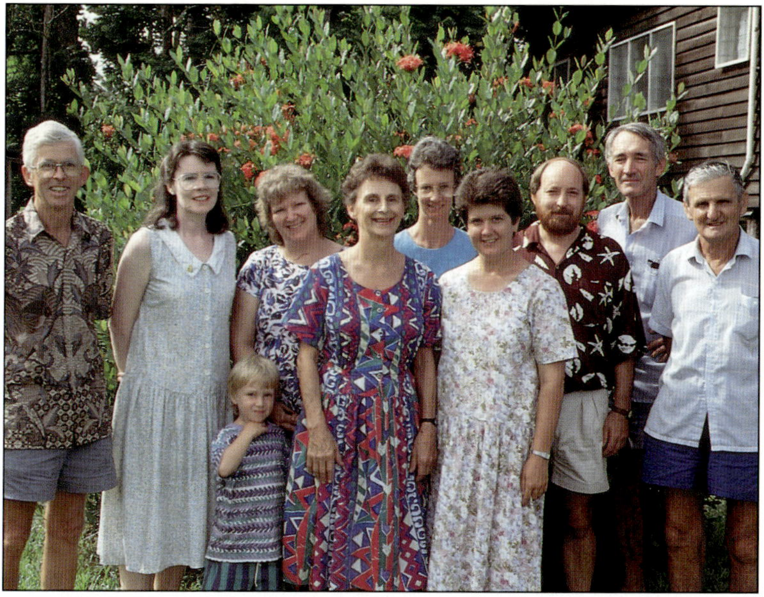

Left: Jenny at the pumps, Makapa
Above: Balimo mission team
Below left: Dr Andrew Baur with River Rover 401
Below right: Jean Goodman, River Rover 402

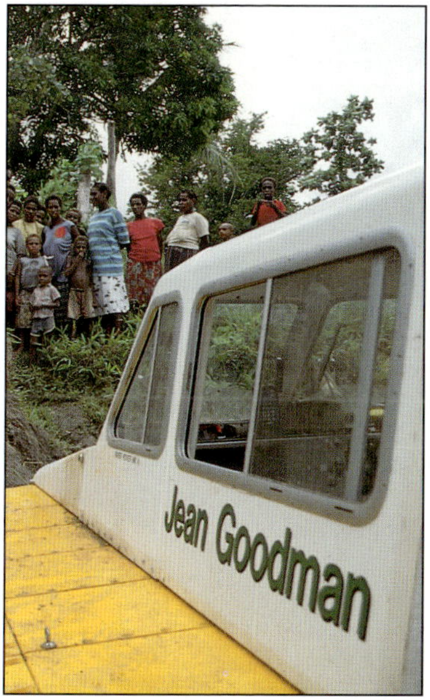

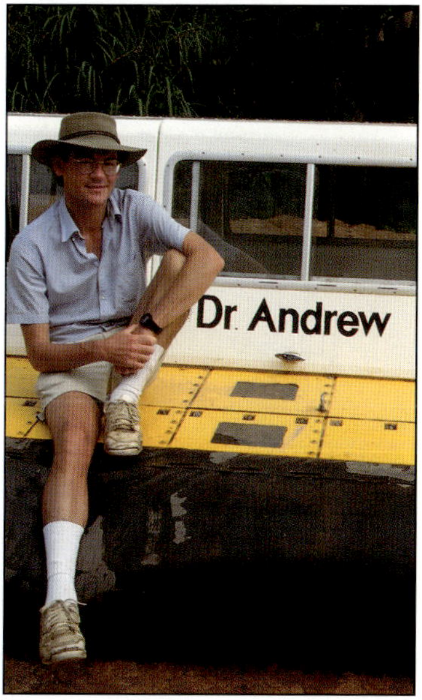

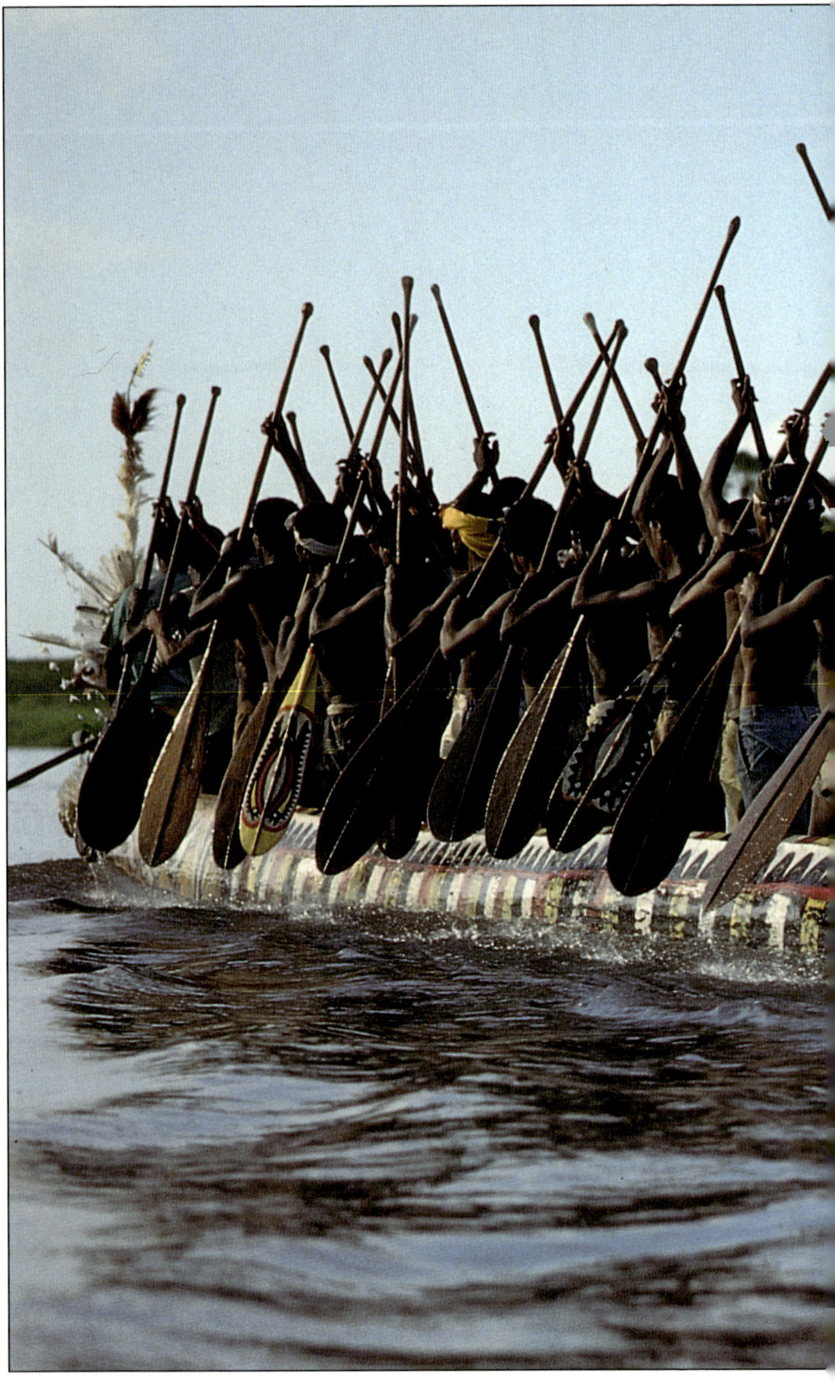

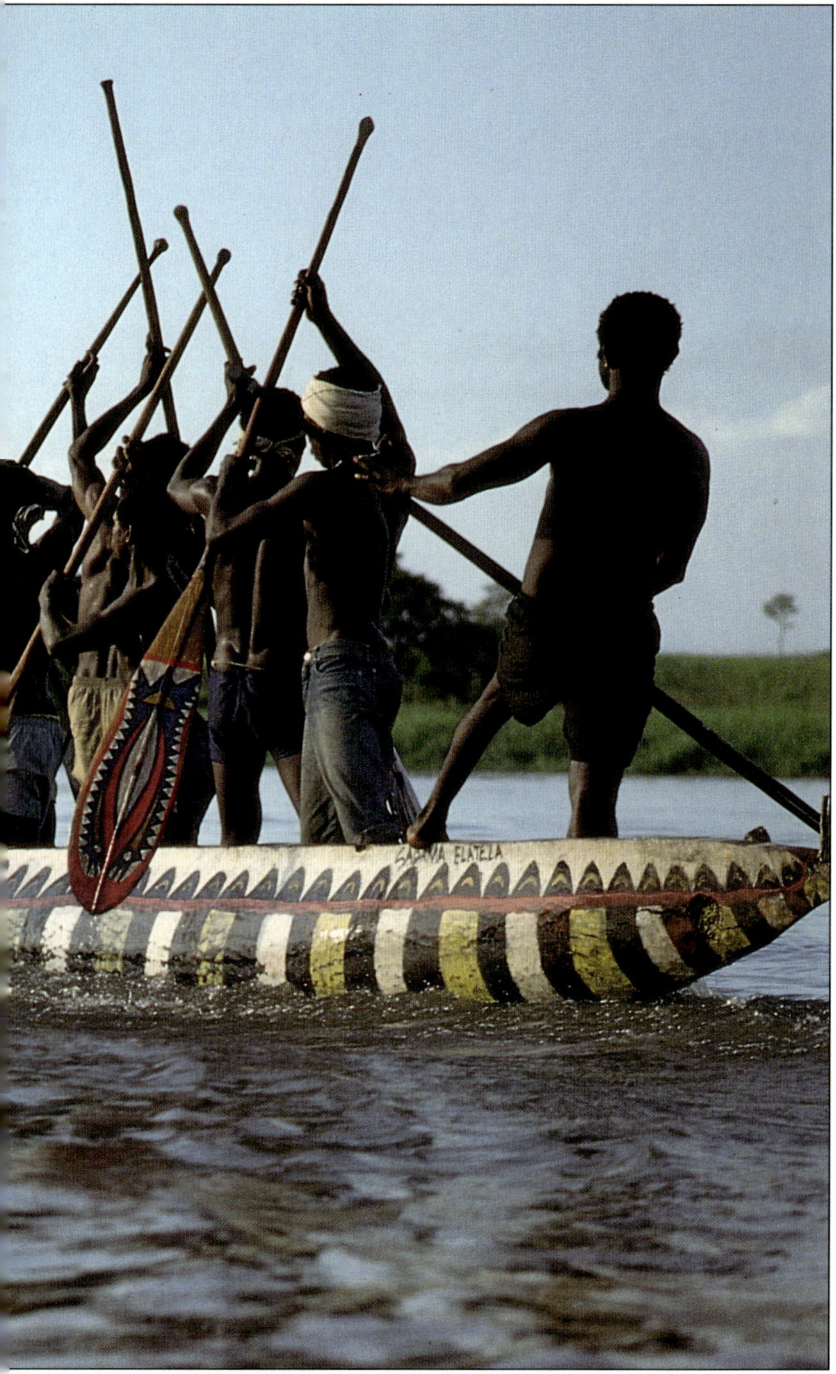
ELATELA

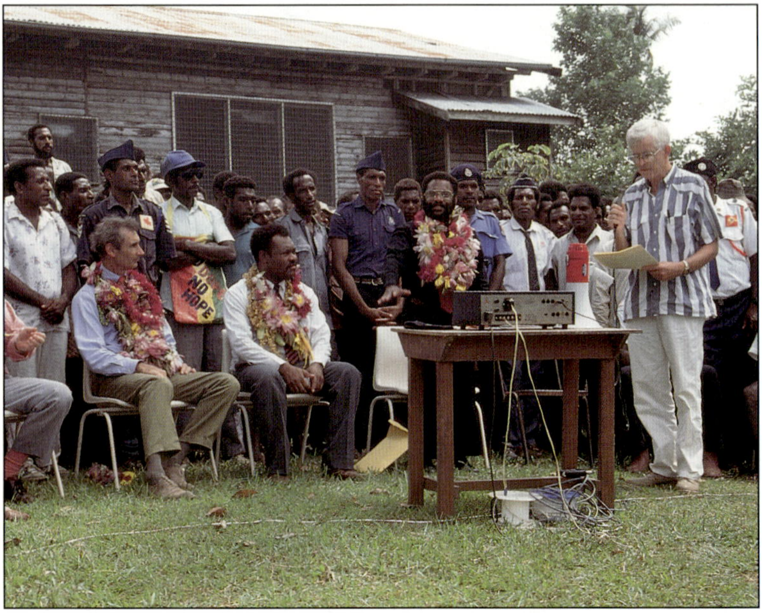

Above: 5 May 1993, handover to Dr Graham Tucker
Below: All join the celebration
Previous page: Gogodala racing canoe in action

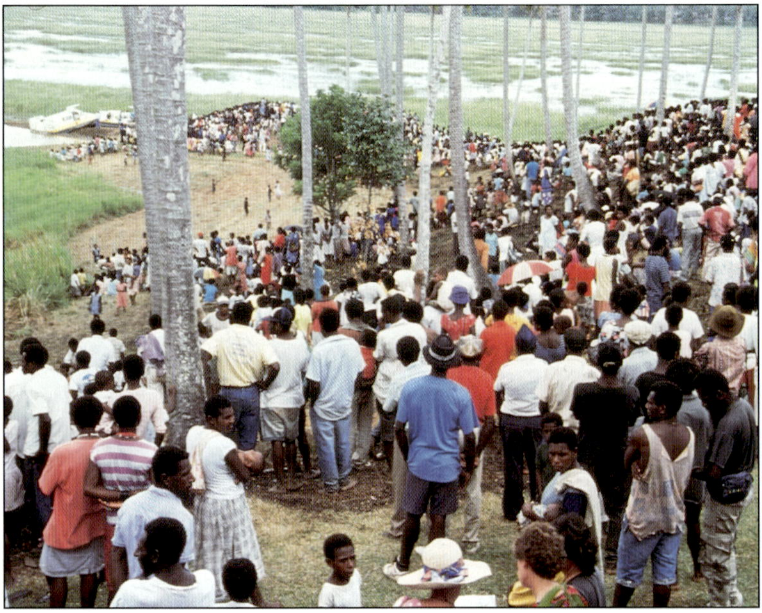

sleep. In the past, each village had a single longhouse in which the whole community lived. Now, as the largest building in the village, the church seems to have replaced some of the communal functions of the longhouse. The floor retains the traditional earth fireplaces which are used regularly, and often the building is used as a guesthouse. On more than a few occasions our female doctors and medical students found themselves, somewhat inappropriately, sharing a church overnight with the local rugby team. On enquiring, they were told, 'When the boys want to "fight" to win, they leave their wives for a few nights and sleep together in the church. They build up their strength for the game.' That used to be the practice before a raiding party would go off to storm a neighbouring village on a payback mission or when head hunting.

Food presented no problem. Starting to raid their compo rations, our medical duo soon found themselves treated to village hospitality. Sago appeared, mixed with catfish or barramundi, wrapped in banana leaves and cooked on the edge of the fires in the floor of the church; there were also giant freshwater prawns. While the meal continued, at the other end of the church the village evening worship service was under way, lit only by hurricane lamps. Small pools of yellow light, dimly lit dark skins merging with the shadows, fires glowing and lighting up darker recesses with flickering flames, cooking smells and singing — the combination created a memorable atmosphere.

Before settling for the night, Ray and Sarah were guided by the nurses in the dark to a small wooden building, the only lavatory for the whole village. Before being taught health education by the patrols, the village had no sanitation, and as a result disease was rife. Even a basic level of sanitation makes a significant difference to the health of a village, particularly when a clean water supply is also provided. Then Ray and Sarah were taken to wash. Stripping off to wash at the edge of the lagoon on a warm, star-spangled night may sound romantic, but there are the mosquitoes to contend with. On their return it was time to set up the bedroll and mosquito net. The nets are wonderful, provided one can ensure that the mossies are on the right side! Sarah got into a terrible muddle and claims she succeeded only in trapping the insects inside. She had an uncomfortable night and awoke to find she had numerous bites. Our medics were experiencing these conditions only briefly, but this is the normal way of life in the villages.

The next morning the patrol held another clinic, again checking on the weight and health of babies and giving immunisations. On then to Makapa, the next stopping point two hours upriver. Prawns and coconut milk on the journey provided lunch, leaving the patrol ready for action on landing at Makapa. It was raining again by the time Makapa was reached, and Ray and Sarah were pleased to unload their kit at the Hendersons where they were to stay overnight. Stuart Henderson is a New Zealander who has lived in PNG for twenty years and his wife Sue was born in Makapa. After a busy clinic seeing more than 200 children, the patrol was treated to a meal prepared by Sue Henderson; later Ray and Sarah enjoyed a conventional shower, the luxury of a bed and falling asleep as heavy rain clattered on the tin roof above.

The patrol moved next morning to Ali, the furthest village up the Aramia reached by the patrols. They had another five hours and more in the canoe, prolonged by taking the wrong creek, the outboard motor failed and they had to paddle the last part of the journey; normal difficulties for these patrols. Ali is an amalgamation of two villages with a population of more than a thousand. Despite its size there is no trained nurse in the village. The only medical service is that provided by the aid post orderly, who has been working there for twenty years. An APO's training is one year shorter than that of a nurse, and so does not attain as high a standard; each year APOs do a two-week refresher course at Balimo. Yet as the only medical service in the village the APO has to deal with many conditions, including caring for nineteen patients with leprosy.

The rain stopped, so it was possible for much of the clinical work, apart from the immunisations, to be done out in the open. The workload was also lighter than at Makapa, so the whole procedure was not as demanding. That night, the Balimo nurses on the patrol took pity on Sarah. After cooking an evening meal the nurses insisted on putting up her mosquito net for her and tucked her in for the night to save her from the depredations of the mosquitoes. As a result she had a good night and was in a better state for the start of the journey back home the next day.

We arrived back from Moresby just before the patrol returned on the afternoon of Good Friday. It was good to be back. I had not realised before how much I had settled in at Balimo; there was almost a sense of returning home. I was glad to have left behind the tensions of the capital. The presence of private security guards, their truncheons dangling, outside supermarkets, the razor-wired condominiums favoured by the expatriate communities, the heavy steel-door grilles of even the ECP houses there, these indicated problems with the 'rascals', the local criminal element. Coupled with the apparent lack of any form of civic pride, an obvious litter problem, notices forbidding the chewing of betel nuts and, in places, the betel-juice-stained pavements, it was obvious that the government has many problems to solve in the capital. By contrast, Balimo is paradise!

Before we had left Balimo for the Port Moresby launch, great progress had been made on the hover-garage. Only a week after laying the last of the concrete floor slabs, the main timber frame had been erected, most of the infilling timber wall panels had been completed and the grading of the 'runway' finished right up to the hover-garage doors. On his final morning before leaving for Moresby, Dick drove RR 401 all the way from the lagoon up to the front of the skeleton building, then manoeuvred the craft inside it. To see the hovercraft housed in its new base for the first time was a significant moment for us. Now, on our return, almost all the roof sheeting was in place, much of the weather boarding was up and the ventilation louvres fixed. It was really encouraging to see. In less than a week the structure had been transformed into a usable building, even though there were still tasks to complete. By the time 402 arrived, the engineers would be able to do servicing and engineering adjustments under cover in the hover-garage.

Jonathan had supervised the packing of the remaining stores and the loading of 402 onto the *Motuan Chief* before he left Moresby. Laurabada were shipping hovercraft and stores out to Balimo for us without charge, as part of the company's continuing support for the expedition. Loaded on a hatch cover, the hovercraft could be lowered over the side directly into the water at Coconut Island near Balimo, rather than being taken all the way over to Kawito. That would save time and we were keen now to have both craft operational so progress could be made in training the national drivers, and with exploration of the wider use of the hovercraft beyond the lagoon where lay their greatest potential for saving lives.

Graeme Bencke, guided by Graham Tucker, had completed the vetting of the original fourteen applicants for the driver training programme. After interviews, eight had been selected for training. They had each been given a brief hands-on introduction to driving, then went through a series of lessons on theory. That had been followed by more driving and practical tests to identify those with the greatest aptitude for handling these unusual vehicles. Eventually the number was whittled down to four, selected for final training to enable them to operate the service after we departed. They would need to be up to standard at least a week before that. On 5 May there was to be an official handover ceremony at Balimo attended by the Minister for Health and the British High Commissioner and it was important to demonstrate the national drivers' ability at that ceremony. They also had to be trained by the engineers so they would be able to maintain the craft.

The Easter weekend came as a very welcome break. Everyone had been working hard and we enjoyed a few days' holiday. Easter, too, was a wonderful reminder of our central purpose in being at Balimo. It gave us a special opportunity to worship with the Christians at Balimo and to demonstrate the bond of faith between us. We started Easter Day by joining a memorable sunrise service out on Mission Point with the missionary doctors, nurses and a number of other Gogodalas from the village. It was a beautiful experience to watch the sunrise as we rejoiced in the fact of the resurrection with the 'Family Bilong God' at Balimo. The occasion conjured up pictures of a wave of sunrise services rolling across the world in a twenty-four-hour celebration of Easter.

We had been invited to take part in the Easter Day service in the English-Speaking Church, and I had been asked to be the speaker. Members of the team under the able direction of Sarah had been rehearsing a dramatised reading of the resurrection story. Hidden talent for mime was revealed by many. There was a great deal of fun in the rehearsals and the performance gave the congregation plenty of amusement, as well as conveying the essential message, evidenced by the response to the appeal to a renewed commitment which Graham Tucker gave at the close of the service. Certainly it was an Easter for us to remember.

By Monday the workers were getting restive and keen to get on with things; there was now only a month to the end of the project and some would be leaving before that. We couldn't afford another day of holiday. Changes were taking place in our routine, too, for several of the team had moved out of our two houses to house sit for some of the doctors and nurses who were going off in rotation to attend one of the ECP Easter conferences. Even in this peaceful place there was a small 'rascal' element, and it was thought unwise to leave furnished houses unoccupied if this could be avoided. Another change would be the arrival of the four-man TV film crew who would be making a video film for the UK's Channel Four and *National Geographic* of America. They would be living and working alongside us for the rest of the project and drawing on some of the material that Jonathan had already filmed.

It was on Thursday evening that things started to go wrong. We had learned about the delays involved in transport arrangements in PNG but we had yet to learn that sometimes arrival could be early. Gareth and Jenny were staying in the Tuckers' house while they were away and so from time to time Gareth heard the 'radio scheds' (regularly timed message sessions). We were not expecting the *Motuan Chief* until Saturday at the earliest, but Gareth received a report from Bruce Olsen in Moresby that the ship was now likely to arrive 'in the early hours' of Friday morning.

There could be trouble unless we had people on hand as the

ship arrived at Coconut Island. It was the nearest place to Balimo that the ship could reach. There was no quay nor other facilities there, just a muddy river bank. We needed to have 402 unloaded over the side of the ship directly into the water. If the captain found no one at Coconut Island he might drop off smaller goods for collection later, but he would not unload the hovercraft, which would then be taken on to Kawito. Unfortunately there was no means of communication with the ship and we did not know what time it might arrive.

There was another possible complication. While in Moresby we had packed a D box, a small steel container, with the remainder of the medical supplies for the hospital at Balimo. Doubts now arose as to whether the container might be dumped at Coconut Island at some unearthly hour if no one were present to say otherwise. It was really needed at Kawito. Only that morning we had stockpiled equipment and baggage there ready to go back in the D box once we had emptied it. The budget was becoming increasingly strained and we had to take maximum advantage of the free transport being provided by Laurabada.

On receiving Gareth's news, Gordon immediately galvanised into a planning meeting to meet the new circumstances. Conflicting ideas were put forward, some more sensible than others. Signal flares were even tested to judge whether they could be used to summon a work party from Mission Point if a watcher were left at the unloading point on Coconut Island. Eventually, in the absence of more definite news, it was decided to assume an early arrival and plan accordingly. Arrangements were made for a reception party to be up and about at an early hour the next day. RR 401 was to go out to Coconut Island to drop off enough of us to deal with unloading and driving the two hovercraft back to Balimo. Some of the engineers had to be available in case of malfunctions on RR 402 after unloading. The film crew were also to be available on standby ready to respond once we had more positive information. They wanted to film the arrival of the ship and the unloading of RR 402. That meant the Sea Rider would be needed too. By the time the confusion and excitement had died down, it was late. There would be some bleary-eyed early starters next morning.

Transport and communications arrangements in the Western Province are complicated. Ship or plane schedules are frequently disrupted by adverse weather conditions, mechanical breakdown or ships missing the tide. Messages often have to be passed indirectly and, as in a Chinese whispers game, they become distorted in the process, as this particular Friday was to prove.

At 5 am, when normally only the usual couple of early risers would be quietly padding about, there were thumps and bangs, the floors of the timber houses shaking as people prepared kit to take with them. Brian Black had to be ready to go up to Kawito by boat to stay overnight or as long as it took to supervise our unloading and repacking arrangements. He had the task of getting medical and other supplies back to Balimo and our heavy kit off to Moresby. The television crew had to assemble their equipment and to carry it down to the boats or hovercraft, ready to get out when needed.

RR 401 went out from the hover-garage before 6.30 am to check on the arrival of the *Motuan Chief* and to position the camera crew ready to film the approach of the ship. Sea Rider followed with the rest of the crew. But there was no sign of the ship. Heavy fog on the river meant that the ship would have been unlikely to make good time. The hovercraft, with Graeme and Gordon on board and two of the film crew, stayed at Coconut Island to await the ship, and the rest returned in Sea Rider for breakfast.

Our normal 7 am breakfast was enlivened by static-distorted radio messages over the film crew's VHF radios. Speculation was rife as we tried to make sense of the ship's failure to arrive. Then the broken contact was restored with Mapodo, and we learned that the ship had still not passed there on its way upriver. It could not possibly be at Coconut Island before the afternoon at the earliest. Little sympathy was shown for the early risers; one kind soul could not resist letting them know that we were all comfortably seated enjoying breakfast while they sat out in the rapidly rising temperatures. In the confusion, information was passed back to base that the ship had missed the tide over the bar at the mouth of the Bamu River and had been further delayed by fog on the river. This turned out to be pure speculation, source unknown.

What began as situation comedy was rapidly turning into farce. There was another message: RR 401 had broken down and engineers were required to deal with it. A boat was launched with the necessary gear and personnel. Meanwhile, the rest of the team started to go about the other tasks of the day as best they could, while waiting for further news. Jonathan, flying in after seeing the ship off from Moresby, was left kicking his heels for a while at the Balimo airstrip. The tractor and trailer had been chasing backwards and forwards in the chaos and had not been free to collect him until well after he had landed.

Not until lunchtime was further news received. A message had come from Mapodo that the boat had just passed Saiwasi, half an hour downriver from Mapodo. On that basis the ship would arrive at Coconut Island some time after 2.30 pm. So far, it had still not been possible to make contact with the ship, even over the film crew's VHF radio. Nothing more could be done until there was news of the hovercraft.

About half an hour, later they started to trickle in. First arrivals were Chris and Lindsay from the film crew. They were immediately bombarded with questions from all directions. When he could get a word in edgeways, Chris said, 'There's a problem with the fan belts; two have snapped. The hovercraft's being towed into base.'

In a perverse way, this had been a good opportunity for the TV crew to get some action footage of the engineers trying to cope with this new difficulty out on the lagoon.

The news made sense; a couple of days earlier a routine check had shown that the two belts driving the thrust fans were slightly loose and as a result had worn against the pulleys. The severity of the wear was worrying as it indicated undue load on the belts and pulleys. For the moment the engineers were nonplussed as to why. The belts had been tightened up in the hope that all would then be well until the spares arrived on the ship from Moresby. Unfortunately, they had not quite made it.

Everything had been fine until RR 401 was deep in the grass. The crew were taking a short route to the hoverbase. Suddenly there was a complete change of engine note and the craft lurched to one side. Quickly cutting the lift, Gordon 'dumped' the craft in the water and stopped to investigate. The starboard thrust fan was not turning at all. They were deep into grass that was difficult for ordinary boats to penetrate and the crew decided to try reaching open water on one thrust fan alone. The control was hopeless; with one thrust fan out of action, the single fan and rudder could not control the craft's direction. To make matters worse the extra load proved too much for the remaining fan, and the belts on that also broke. They were stranded.

At this point it would have been sensible to radio for help, but the craft did not have an operational radio. The authorities in Port Moresby had refused to license the standard marine band radios we had fitted, despite the fact that they were in general use in much of the rest of the world. A licence could not be issued, they said, unless a complete circuit diagram and list of components were submitted, together with a fee of K1000 (about £750). They insisted on a full evaluation by PNG technicians of these already well-proven sets. The alternative was to select a different radio already approved by the authorities. As trading in or selling the current sets and buying new would be much cheaper than paying the licence fee, we decided to change over the sets. But that could not be done until we were in Moresby at the end of the expedition; in the meantime, there was no means of summoning help in an emergency.

Because the lift fan was separately driven, the hovercraft still had cushion pressure and could hover but it had no means of steering. The answer was to take advantage of the lift and tow the craft with Sea Rider to get it back to base. It was an awkward return.

Steve Moody was next to arrive back. He confirmed the news, but added, 'That's not all. In coming loose the belts have worn one of the pulleys and we'll have to replace it.'

401 was now out of action until the ship arrived, the D box had been unloaded and we could get the spares it contained to Balimo.

This was not a major disaster, but yet another part of getting the craft fully operational in their new environment. It was just as well to find out the snags while the experts were available and the discoveries they made could be relayed to HoverAid on our return as part of further development work. Mechanical devices inevitably go wrong at times. Our role was to prepare the nationals to cope with these problems, and to ensure they had enough spares and technical support. The more difficulties we could deal with during the expedition, the greater would be their knowledge and expertise by the time the team departed.

Nevertheless, we had not anticipated some of the problems we had been experiencing. The engineers increasingly felt that there was some basic and possibly common factor accounting for the difficulties we were finding; so far, it had not been identified. Certainly the pattern was different from previous expeditions.

Thanks to the news from Mapodo, we now had a better idea of the time the *Motuan Chief* was likely to arrive. In the early afternoon the two boats set off, one containing the film crew. Still no sign of the ship. More waiting — impatience showed, as the film crew considered how their time could be better used elsewhere. For want of something to do one of the boats went off downriver for five minutes or so to see if there was any sign of the ship approaching. There was not a glimpse — it really should have arrived by now. Could the wires have been crossed again and the ship have gone direct to Kawito? If so, it would have bypassed the tributary to Balimo. As Brian had to go to Kawito anyway, perhaps it would be best if Jonathan took him there now while the rest waited. Jonathan could then bring back news. The inactivity and the uncertainty were getting through to everyone and action, almost any action, seemed better than just sitting around.

It was only minutes after Sea Rider had gone out of sight around the bend that it reappeared at a great pace with Brian waving frantically and pointing back over his shoulder repeatedly. The red hulk of the *Motuan Chief* followed them into view, towering above the little inflatable boat. The camera crew, who had almost given up hope, now had to position themselves hurriedly to film the unloading. It was 4.30 pm on Friday, a day earlier than the originally scheduled arrival and eight or nine hours later than Gareth's news from Moresby had suggested.

The unloading went off without a hitch. It was duly filmed and everyone set off back to base. There was no point in Brian going off to Kawito now, for the ship would be waiting for a time to unload some other goods at Balimo. As the ship was a day early, no one had yet arrived to unload it. How wise to wait until it was known the ship had definitely arrived before stirring into action, rather than dashing to and fro frenetically dissipating energy.

After unloading, RR 402's performance to Hospital Point was not as good as had been hoped. On the very last 'celebrity run' in Moresby, Steve had noticed a slight drop in performance, but there had not been time to investigate. It was disturbing and only underlined the concern about the power problems of 401.

That same Friday evening Andrew, Ray and I had been invited for supper with Rose and Keith Pauley. They had come out some months earlier from Birmingham, England, to join the ECP mission staff elsewhere in PNG. Then they had been asked to go to Balimo where Keith now taught in the nursing school. Supper at the Pauleys' was a highlight. Using locally available foods, they produced wonderful meals. They also had the gift of presentation, those little touches that turn a good meal into an occasion. A great aid was the bone china dinner service they had shipped out from England, which added a simple elegance to their table. Thomas, their four-year-old son, also played a part in putting guests at ease. He is a bright and articulate boy always ready with questions or some account of his play during the day, often verging on the fanciful, as little boys do. Over coffee we were joined by Celestine, the dean of women at the nursing school. She had offered to take the whole hovercraft group to the church in Balimo village that evening.

We met the rest shortly after leaving the Pauleys'. It was good to have Celestine as a guide; we had not been that way before. Gradually our eyes adjusted to the gloom and we started to marvel again at the stars overhead. Gazing up as we walked, I thought at first I was having a little trouble in focusing my eyes properly. Then I realised that it was not solely the sky I was looking at; there was also a tree covered in fireflies glowing in the dark, like the stars I was admiring. It was fascinating to flick my eyes from tree to sky beyond and back again, comparing the two: the power of the light reaching us from the stars and the delicacy of the insects and their little glow.

A quite different experience awaited us when we arrived at the village church in Balimo. We had been invited to go along to one of the meetings held there every evening. It was conducted in Gogodala, but we welcomed the experience. The meeting was already in progress when we arrived. Quietly taking off our shoes at the back of the church, we moved forward to fill gaps. Cross-legged on the floor, we looked around. The only lighting was from hurricane lamps and a single gaslight over the platform. In the soft light we could see that it was a congregation of all ages. The men were seated on one side, the women on the other. Clearly we were a source of interest to the youngsters, who grinned shyly at us. The singing was rhythmic and harmonious, moving, even though we could not understand a word. It was strangely easy to join in worship despite the language barrier. After all, it was the same God we were praising.

The previous evening, Thursday, Celestine had been our guest at supper in Patterson's. I was sitting next to her and during the meal, in her typically quiet way, she asked if I would pass on an invitation to the team. The villagers in Balimo were inviting us to walk around to the village on Saturday afternoon and use their dugout canoes. This was a wonderful opportunity, as we had been itching to have a go in these simple but effective boats. Celestine also said there might be a surprise for us.

The village looked quite different when we walked through it in daylight on the Saturday afternoon. Celestine, who was again leading us, asked us to pause as we came to the church. Leaving us waiting outside she went in; intrigued, we heard whispers and giggles and then Celestine came out again and said with a grin, 'I think we should go on down to the water.' As we walked across a central grass area between the huts, we seemed to be doing a Pied Piper act as we gathered an increasing crowd. By the time we reached the water's edge we had a large procession behind us. We thought maybe they were looking forward to the fun of seeing us struggling to cope with their very narrow canoes. We had been told that crocodiles were rarely seen in the lagoon but perhaps the Gogodala knew something we didn't, and the odd capsize might provide some drama. Nothing could have been further from their kindly thoughts, of course, as they took good care of us.

Drawn up at the water's edge were a number of the low-sided very narrow canoes the Gogodala use with such skill. We eyed them with a certain amount of misgiving even though it had seemed such a fun idea when we accepted the invitation. Then we noticed two huge canoes being paddled towards us across the water. They had high sides and had been hollowed out from immense logs. Compared with the slim, low-sided canoes these looked like great freighters. As the prows were hauled up on the shore a number of the villagers came out of the crowd behind us, carrying various bundles. They made their way to the large canoes and started to load their bundles in: firewood, pumpkins, bananas, sago, coconuts, the procession of people seemed endless. Puzzled we looked on. I turned to Celestine.

'I don't understand,' I said. 'Where are they taking all this? What's going on?'

'They're for you, for the team,' said Celestine. 'These people want to thank you for what you are doing, for the hovercraft you are giving and all the work you have been doing. It's their way of thanking you.'

We were overwhelmed by their kindness; these people did not have much but they were determined to share with us what they had. And we had come over just to play with their canoes! Before doing so, we had to express our gratitude. Asking Celestine to translate for me, I used the stern of one of the large canoes as a perch and gave a little speech to thank them for their kindness. It was only as I turned around to face the bank on which the people had gathered that I realised just how many were there. The whole village must have turned out to thank us, and it was very touching.

Next we were loaded into the large canoes ourselves, with at the prow one of the local pastors, then a team member, followed by another of the village men and so on, alternately down the canoe until about fifteen were aboard. The second canoe was loaded in similar fashion with all the gifts at our feet. Large paddles more than two metres long were handed to us and the canoes were pushed off. It was to be a race from the spit on which the village is located across the lagoon to the next spit at Mission Point. With grunts and shouts we tried with varying degrees of success to follow the lead and style of our hosts. They made it look so easy! One canoe established a lead. Despite the efforts of the second crew the first only consolidated their lead and amidst great cheering made it to Mission Point first. Not quite the Oxbridge boat race, but it was great fun, thanks to the folk from Balimo.

10

Dedicated Doctors, Logs and Frogs

GRAHAM ZERK'S RETURN TO Balimo as an expedition member was an important event for many people, and they turned out in style to welcome him. There was a good crowd at the airfield as he arrived — former patients, parents with the children he had helped bring into the world, nurses who had worked with him. The floral necklace they put around his neck expressed more than words the regard they had for him. Few doctors would get such a greeting after an absence of two years.

As a twenty-two-year-old medical student Graham Zerk came to Balimo in 1978 for three months of training. Eight years later, a qualified and experienced doctor, he returned to Papua with a wife and four children. At that time Graham Tucker was already medical superintendent at Balimo and the two Grahams were to serve together at the health centre for nearly six years until the Zerk family left to return to Queensland in 1991. During that period another medical student, Andrew Baur, came out to Balimo for a short period of training in late 1988. By September 1990, he too was back as a qualified doctor. All three have a special place in the Balimo hovercraft story.

During his time as a student in Papua New Guinea, Graham Zerk made a particular study of the medical patrols on the Aramia River. He also carried out a survey of the River Wawoi as far as the Wawoi Falls and the length and breadth of the Fly River delta. His sailing and medical interests combined in that work, and from it grew his deep concern for the tribes of the area. When he returned in 1986 he quickly found that the work of the area already being served from Balimo was so demanding that there was no capacity to extend it further, despite the great need. It was all that he and Graham Tucker could do to cope with the existing hospital work and the patrols. But the needs beyond did not go away and there was concern that the Tabo tribe, living downriver from Saiwasi on the edge of the range of the Balimo work, could ultimately become extinct if they did not get a primary health care and medical service. That crisis has not diminished. The need is still greater.

Graham took me by boat to the village of Garu on the Aramia just beyond Saiwasi. Six years ago there were no children in that village under the age of five. Eighty per cent of the women were infected with one or more sexually transmitted diseases, there was no fresh water supply in the village and no means of dealing with sewage or other wastes. Today after six years' contact with the medical patrols from Balimo, the people are just installing their first fresh water supply, a storage tank collecting rainwater from a single corrugated-iron roof over the house of the local headmaster. There is basic drainage but no sanitation to speak of; a building has been put up for an aid post, but as yet there is no orderly to service it. Conditions are improving there, but they still have a way to go, and this is one of the better villages in the area. It is better because it has been brought within reach of the Balimo patrols who can tell the people about the importance of clean water and basic sanitation; better also because the Maternal Child Health programme is under way and because the treatment is available for the serious cases, such as that of the thirteen-year-old boy whose leprous foot Graham examined after the boy took off the filthy rags binding it. He promised that on one of the hovercraft trips the boy would be taken to Balimo for further surgical treatment. The boy then promptly put on the rags again so he could hobble on the remains of his foot to take the doctor across the slimy mud to a hut where, he said, there was a sick woman; so keen was he that others should also benefit from the skill of the doctor. Sadly, when we got there the woman refused to see the doctor. This was not unusual, Graham told me; building up confidence takes a long time.

Elsewhere on the river there were people who greeted 'Jerk' (as they pronounced Graham's surname) as a long-lost friend; there were hugs and slaps, great grins galore, genuine pleasure at seeing again one of those dedicated doctors who had made it their business to care for those who seemed the concern of no one else. Some of the young boys and girls got special greetings from Graham for, as he explained to me, 'I remember bringing that one into the world.' When we went into any village, even in passing, Graham always asked, 'Are there any sick?' This inevitably brought out a crowd for an open-air surgery, with most of the village as an interested audience. Sick babies were laid on the raised balcony floor of a hut to be examined, villagers came forward with various complaints. It was done as a matter of routine because the doctor was there.

It was to work like this that Andrew Baur was attracted. Born in Philadelphia USA, from the age of ten Andrew had wanted to be a missionary. He feared he might never realise that dream for at the age of three he had been diagnosed as diabetic. That did not prevent him enrolling for medical school or asking to train in PNG during his final year. He reasoned that if God could keep him alive there for those two months, there was no reason why he could not do so for three years. Despite that strong commitment his faith was put to the test. During those two months in PNG he suffered eye problems due to the diabetes and had problems with the healing of skin ulcers and cuts for the same reasons. These were more than enough to put the average young man off for life, but not Andrew, who returned to America to finish his training more determined than ever to put that training to good use in PNG. While completing that training he was diagnosed as having a diabetes-related kidney disorder that would eventually require dialysis or a kidney transplant; he also suffered recurring eye problems. Realising that his time for missionary work was going to be limited by his deteriorating health he gave up the general practice work he was doing and applied at once to work in Balimo where, in 1990, he went into the missionary service he had so longed for.

In 1988, while Andrew Baur had been doing his medical training with the two Grahams, the idea of using hovercraft there was growing. It had been around for a little while, but during that time the idea started to expand. But it was not until some time after Andrew's return to the USA that real progress was made. Graham Zerk's father-in-law, a GP in north Queensland, saw an article written by Bill Gould about the Peru expedition. That article fired their imagination for PNG. Eventually, through Helen Brackenbury, contact was established with Mike Cole.

There were, of course, two major problems — manpower and money. By 1989 Graham Zerk's time in PNG was running out. He knew he would be leaving in a little over a year and that just was not long enough to take on the commitment of a hovercraft project. Knowing of Andrew Baur's interest in working in Balimo, Graham contacted Andrew in the States and asked if he would come out to be a 'hover doctor'. Readily Andrew agreed and Graham went ahead and promoted the idea. Without the assurance of Andrew's interest, the idea could not have been developed and translated into reality. Little did they know that Andrew's time at Balimo was going to be even shorter than he had thought. By late 1991, ill health forced his return to the USA. Yet his willingness to be involved was integral to the development of the concept and by the time he had to leave the proposal was well on the way. Through the generosity of his father, Philip Baur, substantial financial backing was raised for the project from the USA, so giving the project a foundation for further fundraising. Andrew has since been able to return to medical work in PNG but in the cooler climate of Wapenamanda in the Enga Province. While his part has been that of a catalyst rather than a participant, he has been remembered for his courage and dedication in the face of his health problems by one of the hovercraft, RR 401, being named the *Dr Andrew*.

The main burden of seeing the project right through its birth pangs fell to Graham Tucker, who had been in from the very beginning. Without his support and enthusiasm, the hovercraft would never have reached Balimo. He came to Balimo originally to set up a surgical department; on that depended the nursing school which has since gone from strength to strength. With the arrival of the hovercraft, he now takes over the operation of another valuable service. It will give this man of quiet strength yet more responsibility which, characteristically, he seems very ready to shoulder. Despite his willingness, he very much needs some help with the day-to-day maintenance work of the hospital. The oversight of the hovercraft service only creates an extra load for an already very busy doctor.

Now we had the second hovercraft, it was time to explore the day-to-day implications of using the craft for patrols and emergency journeys. But first we had to get our spares off the *Motuan Chief*, for we needed 401 back in service. Without it the training of the selected national drivers could not continue at the required pace.

Although Brian had gone off to Kawito on the Saturday, the ship itself did not arrive until the Sunday. There had been yet another delay at Coconut Island awaiting the unloading of cargo for Balimo. Had we known, we would not have been concerned about our own items being dumped there unattended. Brian had no problems over locating and unpacking the D box nor repacking it with our heavy gear for the return journey. The urgently needed spares and some food supplies were more troublesome. Because they were needed first these items had been packed separately on a pallet for ready access. Jonathan had ensured that they were loaded, and their recovery should have been straightforward; but it wasn't. The pallet could not be found. Brian had hours of slow dehydration while searching vainly in the oven temperature of the ship's hold, and enduring the diesel fumes from a forklift truck used for unloading. The ensuing radio sequence as he passed the news on an open channel was confused.

'Brian Black for Gordon Goodman, over.'

'Gordon here, Brian, go ahead, over.'

'The pallet's not on the ship, over.'

'What d'you mean, it's not on the ship? Jonathan saw it loaded! Over.'

'I said,' (was that gnashing teeth or static?) '*it's - not - on - the*

- ship, over!'

'Brian, it's got to be there. You'll just have to look again. Could it have been unloaded and put away somewhere in one of the sheds without your realising? Over.'

A long, long, pause ...

'Balimo, Kawito, are you receiving? Over.' It was Gordon again, as there was no reply.

'Yes, Gordon, I'm receiving! Okay, I'll try again, but it's just not here. It's not even listed on the ship's manifest. You'll have to contact Laurabada tomorrow and find out what they've done with it. Over.'

'Okay, Brian. Have another search, and if it really is not there let me know and I'll contact them. Happy searching. Out.'

There were more explosions from the loudspeaker, which *might* have been static.

The news was received with total disbelief. There was frustration at the non-arrival of the essential spares, not to mention our desperately needed breakfast cereal. Understandably, on his return empty-handed on the Monday, Brian did not think us at all appreciative of what he had been through. Nevertheless, he was adamant that the pallet had *not* been on the ship; at least he was until the message was received from the Laurabada office, firmly stating that the pallet had definitely been loaded on the ship. Now we were really concerned; by then the ship had left Kawito and was on its way downriver heading back to Moresby. Unless it could be intercepted, the whole process of getting the goods from Moresby would have to be started again and that would take weeks.

As Graeme Bencke brought 402 in to Mission Point after a morning spent training the national drivers, he could see Gordon waiting on the shore.

'The pallet was on the *Motuan Chief* all the time!' Gordon said. 'We're going to have to chase the ship down the river. Grab some lunch and get a crew together. I want you to get off as soon as you can. There's no time to waste.'

'How far's the ship gone, Gordon?'

'I don't know; you'd better take ration packs, emergency kit and overnight equipment with you so you can be ready for anything. We've have just got to have those spares from the pallet.'

Quickly Graeme sorted out who he should take. 'Okay, I'll take Sebia with me. It'll be good training for him. Jonathan could be useful. He'd be able to recognise the pallet. He might be able to do some filming too. Tim could give engineering backup. We don't need more than four of us — it'll keep the weight down anyway.'

After a hasty lunch and refuelling the hovercraft, they set off at a good pace through the lagoon and onto the Aramia. In an hour and a quarter they had passed Mapodo, half the time taken by a canoe with an outboard. Without stopping they pressed on with all speed, hoping to sight the red hulk of the *Motuan Chief* round every bend. The contrast as they reached the mouth of the Aramia was stark; instead of the confining tree-lined banks of the twisting river, the Bamu stretched out before them, seemingly immense. Still there was no sign of the ship.

There was nothing for it but to head upriver for Emeti, the next calling point for the ship. This was the farthest the hovercraft had been taken, so valuable experience was being gained, even as they pursued what was starting to seem like an elusive ship. As the empty jetty came into sight they could feel the disappointment and concern mounting. How much further were they going to have to travel; would they have enough fuel? The hovercraft was beached on the narrow mud bank, to the great excitement of the crowd that had appeared out of nowhere as the hovercraft came into earshot. Sebia was able to find out that at midday, before they had even left Balimo, the ship had pulled out from Emeti to travel even further upriver to Kamusi on the Guari, a tributary of the Bamu. A conference led to the decision to attempt a quick dash upriver to Kamusi to rescue the urgently needed parts. It should then be possible to get back as far as Mapodo by nightfall.

But they were reckoning without technical problems. Pulling away from Emeti, Jonathan noticed a flapping skirt finger. Once again it was at the rear nearside corner of the craft, apparently a vulnerable position. Under the pressure of time they decided to press on. Within a short distance, however, six more fingers were loose in the same area; the loss of lift as a result made it impossible to keep speed over hump, battle though they might. There was no alternative but to beach and effect a repair — but where? By now the banks of the Bamu were heavily forested down to the water's edge with no margin for beaching. It took some time at their reduced speed before a tiny bank was found. Less than half the hovercraft could be beached leaving the damaged rear corner in the water. Jonathan, otherwise known as 'Fingers Allan', stripped off to the bare essentials to get into the murky water while the others kept a sharp lookout for crocodiles; we had heard enough well-documented accounts to know that the risk was a very real one. Infrequent though their appearances were, they could be dramatic and safety could not be taken for granted. In the darkness under the hull and the skirt, Jonathan had to do most of the work by touch, struggling to keep his footing on the slimy mud. Before the repairs were completed the supply of spare bolts ran out. Improvising, a couple of bolts were taken out of one of the rear door hinges to complete the job.

It was two hours before the repairs were completed and they could get under way again. The mission would have to be abandoned as they could not take the risk of further damage stranding them altogether. They headed back down the Bamu and into the mouth of the Aramia. It was important to contact Balimo but that could not be done from Emeti, as the radio link didn't reach that far. The best they could do would be to get as far as Mapodo before dark and radio from there to let Gordon know the position. In future larger supplies of spare bolts must be carried; this was one of the earliest lessons learned. Also, while the shear bolts correctly protected the skirt fingers, it would be necessary to decide whether they were of the right strength. If they were, there had to be some other reason why skirt fingers were pulling out so readily.

RR 402 was now going well again and with some confidence they decided that it would be possible to reach Mapodo before nightfall. But they were travelling upriver against a strong current. The light was failing fast when they were still some distance from Mapodo. They pressed on at full speed as long as they dared, keeping a sharp lookout for the heavy waterlogged tree trunks that, almost totally submerged, floated downstream with the current. It would be easy in the poor light to miss seeing one and even a passing blow could rip out the side of the skirt and strand them altogether in the darkness leaving them drifting helplessly.

It was just dark enough to start using the halogen hand lamp to scan the river ahead for obstacles. As Jonathan reached for the lamp a darker shadow loomed immediately ahead. 'Look out!' he yelled. Graeme slammed the right elevons closed and opened the throttle fully in a desperate attempt to swerve to the right, away from the submerged log. The full force of the current was thrusting it directly at the hovercraft like a massive battering ram as the two collided. The impact wrenched River Rover round to the left, throwing the crew off balance as, with immense power, the tree trunk was swept inexorably on by the current. Rotating fully, the craft was now facing downriver, drifting helplessly in midstream as Graeme closed the throttle and shut the elevons. There, floating away from them, visible in the beam of the lamp, was the log, followed by a section of the foam from the underside of the craft. With an effort they retrieved the foam and then took stock of their position.

Graeme's last-minute swerve had avoided a head-on collision but as it swept down the left-hand side of the craft, the log had torn out a number of fingers. The last of the bolts had been used in the repairs on the Bamu, so there were no more left for repairs even if the crew had been able to see well enough in the light of their only lamp. Opening up the engine again, Graeme tentatively explored what performance remained. Try as they might, there was not enough lift from the damaged skirt to get the craft over hump speed. Even if there had been, continuing might result in a repetition of the crash, only making the position worse. As they pondered their dilemma, a dim light was seen approaching from downriver. It was an outboard-powered canoe making its way upriver by the dim light of a torch. Sebia hailed the canoe and with the help of its willing crew the hovercraft was towed into the bank and roped to some trees. Hitching a lift from their rescuers, they intended to get as far as Waia village. From there Sebia was confident he could guide them in the dark through the jungle to Mapodo which lay on the other side of an isthmus in a sweep of the river.

Within minutes another canoe appeared from upriver. The noise of the impact with the log had been heard by Tim Schlatter, who with his wife Karen and their children lived only half a mile (a kilometre) or so from where the collision had occurred. Help was at hand, just when it was most needed. Tim worked among the Tabo tribe and for five years had been making the first written version of their language and then translating it. The Tabo translation of St Mark's Gospel we had heard read in the college at Mapodo was the result of Tim's work. Earlier in the day the Schlatters had seen the hovercraft going downstream and had been expecting its return. They had heard the noise of the approaching hovercraft, then the impact, followed by the efforts to get over hump and finally silence, and Tim Schlatter set out to investigate.

Relaxing at the Schlatters' home, the hovercraft crew contrasted their surroundings with their anticipated night in the stranded craft with only a mosquito net and compo rations for creature comforts, or walking through the jungle on a narrow track with the dim light of one small torch as the only means of defence against poisonous snakes. They were now being very well looked after. Tim Schlatter managed to get an explanatory radio message through to Balimo; he also requested spares. The crew had only to relax and wait.

But the radio exchange provided an exasperating piece of news. The pallet of goods had been located at Kawito. Unknown to Brian, it had been taken off the ship before his arrival so the chase had been in vain. Because it was unlabelled the pallet had been placed in the back of one of the sheds for someone to claim it. Unfortunately, no one had thought to tell Brian. How it came to be on the ship but not on the ship's manifest remains a mystery. However, though the hovercraft crew's journey had been unnecessary, they had gained some eventful operational experience. At least the much-needed spare parts had been found.

Looking a little pathetic, 402 was towed to Saiwasi by canoe next morning, ready for repairs to the skirt once the spares arrived. Any further examination for greater damage would have to wait until the craft could be raised on the newly installed lifting tackle in the base building at Balimo. By lunchtime, RR 401 arrived with Gordon and Ben aboard and the spares. Within half an hour the repairs had been done and both craft were on their way back.

One river dash was over, but there was another to come. First, though, we had to deal with the frogs.

In an area where the number of frogs exceeds the human population by many hundreds, if not thousands, frogs are bound to appear at times where they are not wanted. Given that water is their natural habitat, we might have anticipated what happened. Several days must have passed before the problem was really identified. There had been the occasional reference to the taste of the water but most of us had not been overly concerned. Only when turning on the water tap in Patterson's produced a distinctly unpleasant smell did it become obvious that something was really wrong. The water was declared unsafe for drinking. It was unacceptable for washing too, which meant that the tank at Lagoon View was the only source of good water. There had been no rain for some days, so the supply levels were not high. In a climate where dehydration is a constant threat this was a potentially serious position. Quantity apart, it was also an inconvenience. All the cooking, eating and much of the drinking was done in Patterson's and now every drop of water had to be carried over in buckets and jugs from the other house.

The water supply came from two large circular tanks. Rainwater from the tin roofs was fed into the tanks through a gauze sieve. One of the tanks was set up high on posts like the houses, and from it water flowed by gravity to the taps in the house. In the dry weather we had been having, water had been rationed at times while we waited for the next heavy rain. In our densely populated houses we needed huge quantities of water to keep us going.

Martin Healey drew the short straw and was given the job of tank clearance contractor. First the problem had to be identified. That meant climbing up to examine the upper tank. The access lid was taken off. There, floating in the water, was a large dead frog. As soon as an improvised net touched it, the frog disintegrated into a fine powder across the surface of the maturing brew we had been drinking for no one knew how many days! What might be termed retrospective hypochondria soon set in. Despite the loss of water it would involve, the tank had to be emptied and cleaned. Eventually this was completed and the tank disinfected. All we could do now was to continue being economical with the water, pray for rain and hope for strong stomachs.

After the log encounter the engineers needed to see what damage had been done to the hovercraft, a difficult job had it not been for the lifting beam we had erected. Setting the lifting beam up had been a daunting job and Gareth, an immensely practical man, had prepared for it carefully. Three steel beams had to be bolted together in an inverted U shape and the legs dropped into two deep holes ready for concrete to be poured around them. We had no crane or other heavy lifting tackle to do the job for us, so it had to be muscle power, aided by Tim on the tractor. Bolting the steel together on the ground was no problem, apart from a bit of weight lifting. The ends of the legs lay nicely over the holes they had to drop into. But how to get them upright in the holes? With enough of us lifting, we could get the top beam up to waist height but that was as far as we could go. By hooking the end of the tractor lifting arm under the top beam and standing clear, we could get it up another yard (metre) or so, but no further. At that point the ends of the legs started to slide into the waiting holes at a shallow angle but their weight made them dig into the boards we had placed upright in the holes.

We stood back and thought. The situation did not look promising. There was a long way to go and we had used up all our lifting ability. We did have hauling power, that was what a tractor was for. Then an idea came. Tim tied several of the Phantom aeroplane straps between the tractor and the beam. They had not been strong enough for a straight lift of the hovercraft, but they should do this job.

As the tractor took up the slack, the steel moved slowly upwards. Carefully the props were repositioned to hold the gains we had made if anything snapped or slipped; the bottom of the legs dug ever more deeply into the boards in the holes. The thing was starting to look possible. Encouraged, we went at the remaining pull with a will, hauling on ropes to help the tractor.

With a sudden lurch, the whole steel assembly slid down to the bottom of the holes and stood almost upright. Giving one of his famous war whoops, Gareth jumped up and down in triumph, and we cheered and yelled with him. Brawn, brain and a little machine help had triumphed; maybe we were starting to really tune in to the PNG way of doing things rather than relying solely on Western technology. After that, the rest was easy: we simply had to set the uprights truly vertical and set the legs in concrete.

Now the engineers were able to use the strong beams to lift up the hovercraft and examine the underside of the fibreglass hull to see what damage the log impact had caused. Part of the skirt diaphragm was torn, there was some minor impact damage to the hull and a bend in one of the metal sections which ran the length of the fibreglass hull to strengthen it. None of the damage was of immediate concern, which was reassuring. No matter what care was taken in normal operational use, there would inevitably be incidents like this when the craft were in regular use on the rivers. At least the experience had shown that the structure was robust enough for the job. Meantime, 402 could go back into service and the repairs could wait for a convenient break in the driver training and exploration programme.

The next foray was westward in preparation for a possible pioneering drive to find a route between the Aramia and the Fly. If that could be found, the potential for improving the access to the villages on the north banks of the mid-Fly would be considerable. It might prove possible to go the long way round via the Bamu and south into the mouth of the Fly delta, but the logistics of fuelling on the journey and coping with the sheer scale of the tides, winds and the massive water flow out through the mighty delta were enormous. If a shorter western route could be found there could be great advantages.

First some planning had to be done and fuel dumps established along the Aramia. While doing an early recce for that, it might be possible to explore the creek to Pikawa north of the Aramia on the western side of Awaba. It would also be a good opportunity to call in at Awaba and replenish our dwindling meat stocks. Russell Peake, an ECP agriculturalist, had established a modest cattle station there and was encouraging the Gogodala in the area to take cattle on agistment. In return for grazing and caring for a number of the cattle station beasts for two years, a man would be given a cow and a calf so he could start to build up his own small herd. An abattoir had been built at Awaba and meat was supplied to the surrounding area, so a market for the product was building up. The individual small farmers could use the Awaba abattoir as a marketing co-operative for their cattle. It was a good scheme, gradually offering the means of increasing the area's earning capacity.

The intended Pikawa trip was not a success; in fact, the attempt was abandoned. It did, however, reveal some information that assumed significance later. From early on, RR 402 was not performing well. The first setback came as the craft turned west out of the lagoon. Progress was extremely slow against a strong headwind, embarrassingly so when the hospital dinghy appeared alongside. It had left Balimo after the hovercraft, and here it was, about to overtake. Something was not right. For the moment nothing could be done, apart from lightening the load, so one of the passengers bound only for Kawito was transferred to the dinghy. That helped and Kawito was reached without incident, but performance was sluggish and no better than the dinghy at any time.

On the way to Awaba Graeme Bencke took the opportunity to extend driver training on the finer points of hovercraft turns. Martin Fairley, who was driving, enthusiastically attempted an ambitious turn in the river. The result was exciting and more than he, and certainly his passengers, expected. No one is quite sure what happened. The hovercraft made a startling swing around and finished up facing in the direction opposite from that intended. Once the excitement had died down they got on their way again but performance was, if anything, even more sluggish.

Arriving at Awaba part of the reason became clear; six skirt finger tie-bolts had been broken, possibly due to the stress of the dramatic turn. Again the damage was on a rear corner. The fingers were coming off in those areas far too easily for comfort. The craft was beached and repairs were made. As they were finishing, Gareth appeared. The MAF pilot landing at Kawito had seen from the air that 402 was in trouble and had passed the news on to Gareth. Like a river equivalent of the Automobile Association, he had come along to help. So much time had been taken up by the poor performance and repair that it was decided to abandon the idea of reaching Pikawa on this trip.

With a tail wind the return journey went better but there was clearly something wrong. The reason was not hard to find once 402 was hoisted up in the workshop. Dangling from the underside of the hull was a large sheet of the closed cell foam used to cushion impact. As it dragged in the water, it had been causing considerable resistance and so significantly reducing power. Although the importance of that discovery was not immediately recognised, it did hold the clue to a general improvement in performance that was achieved later. But the extra drag alone did nothing to explain why fingers pulled loose so easily.

While the craft was up, the engineers repaired the damage from the log impact. Brute force straightened the aluminium skeg, the strengthening strip on the underside of the hull — Gareth lay on his back under the hull wielding a heavy sledgehammer. Just his sort of job! Trustingly, Graeme Benke held the piece of wood that Gareth was hammering against the metal strip. Resin and glass fibre healed the hull itself and patches and adhesive mended the rip in the skirt diaphragm. Each operation gave valuable experience to the Gogodala trainees. The ability to carry out these repairs would be essential for day-to-day operation of the hover ambulance service; the ease with which it could be done with limited skills and facilities was an essential feature of the hovercraft design. Now that we were forming a good appreciation of the things that could go wrong, the time had come to start to push out the boundaries a little. Performance still had to be improved, and the engineers would carry on working on that, but more testing still had to be done. There were also more sombre hospital duties to be performed.

11

All in a Night's Work

DEATH IS NEVER MORE poignant than when it claims a young child. The hovercraft were being provided to help save life and, obvious though it is, we had not thought much about them being involved with death; certainly not that of a young child. Jonathan and Gareth were brought starkly face to face with such a tragedy when Gordon gave them an assignment. A nine-year-old girl suffering from acute of malaria had been brought to the hospital by her parents from beyond Emeti. Unfortunately, it had not been possible to save her life. Now there was the sad task of returning the body and the grieving parents to their home.

The body of the child was brought down to the hover-garage in the hospital ambulance. Although completely wrapped in white plastic, its shape was clearly distinguishable as they laid it on the folded-down seats of the hovercraft. The diminutive size of the package evoked feelings of deep sadness and helplessness as it lay down the centre of the hovercraft, the grieving parents sitting on either side. Already, after three days, there was a pungent odour in the tropical heat. With windows wide open they set off on their melancholy journey, the noise of the engine and fans discordant in the presence of death.

Perhaps fittingly, progress was slowed a little by strong headwinds. Little was said on the journey; words hardly seemed appropriate in the face of grief, and the parents spoke little English. With only a brief stop at Mapodo to refuel and to change drivers, the sombre journey continued, until slightly eased for Gareth and Jonathan by the wonder of the Bamu River's vastness as the hovercraft emerged from the mouth of the Aramia and headed upstream. Soon they reached Emeti, where they tried to find out where the parents came from. Their village, it seemed, was some distance from Emeti, beyond the fuel range of the craft. Transport by canoe was arranged for the following day, and with heavy hearts Gareth and Jonathan helped the sorrowful parents out of the craft and carried the pathetically small package up the bank. As they looked back, their last picture was the heart-wrenching spectacle of the grieving family standing helplessly on the bank, surrounded by curious onlookers.

Locked into thoughts of the incident Gareth and Jonathan continued in silence for some time until the failing light recalled matters of more immediate concern. They could not reach Saiwasi before dark; so they had two choices: to moor up and camp on the river for the night, or to wait until it was fully dark and then continue cautiously using the beam of the halogen hand lamp. Jonathan still had vivid memories of crashing into the log a few nights before and was not anxious to repeat the experience. That incident occurred in the half light and they reasoned that it should be possible to proceed with caution in reasonable safety once it was fully dark. They decided to give it a try. With no convenient shelving bank to beach the hovercraft, they could only 'dump' it on a patch of tall reeds while waiting for darkness. The craft was far from secure and three times it was dragged off by the strong flow of the Aramia. A passing canoeload of nationals offered to rescue Gareth and Jonathan, thinking they were stranded. Ever ingenious when it came to food, Jonathan found an innovative use for his tiny butane flame soldering iron. It could double effectively as a stove, for heating tins of food from the compo rations; eating helped to pass the time while they waited.

Moonlight was the last thing they wanted. The soft light reduced the contrast between the lamp beam and darkness, making it less easy to pick out obstructions on the river. But they could not wait for cloud forever and the sky might stay clear all night. So with Gareth outside on the decking at the front of the craft holding the hand lamp, Jonathan took 402 forward at no more than seven or eight knots, just over hump speed. Anxiously he peered ahead along the bright pencil beam that threw everything else into confusing variegated shadow. As they concentrated on the beam, it was very easy to become disorientated in the wide, twisting Aramia. Suddenly, as the river took a sharp bend, Jonathan found he was heading the craft directly for one of the banks. The sudden loss of speed startled Gareth as Jonathan cut the throttle, not knowing whether to turn right or left. Quickly Gareth swung the lamp beam to guide him onto the right track and the craft was turned upstream again. From then on Jonathan decided to follow the right bank of the river closely.

Direct verbal communication between the two of them was difficult with Gareth outside and Jonathan within. As they gingerly felt their way along, a method emerged. Most of the time Gareth kept the beam on the right-hand bank so Jonathan could follow it. Every few seconds he swept the beam across the river ahead. Any obstacle above water, whether a pole or a patch of reeds, was highlighted, throwing a dark shadow on the water behind it; significant obstacles were urgently brought to Jonathan's attention as Gareth flashed the light beam quickly up and down on them. As soon as he detected a response on the controls Gareth turned the beam on the bank again and resumed scanning, occasionally swinging the beam back on the obstacle until it had been safely negotiated.

Their confidence grew as speed increased. By the time they reached Tim Schlatter's house at Saiwasi, it seemed feasible to carry on at least as far as Mapodo. Slowing down only enough to shout their plans to Tim, they pressed on, building up yet more speed until they were travelling through the night at seventeen knots while their technique improved. At that rate it was possible to make Balimo in reasonable time. Changing positions, they decided to press on, taking the chance of finding their way through the lagoon in the dark now they knew it better. Surprisingly, they were not the only craft on the river in the dark. There were many dugouts travelling solely by the light of a hand-held torch, and they had to keep a sharp look out for them also.

It was curiously exhilarating sitting out on the nose of the craft, hurtling forward into the darkness of the tropical night, skimming the bank so closely at times that the skirt would brush up against the reeds. The speed was accompanied by a peppering of small flying insects and the sudden swing of the craft as evasive action was taken around an overhanging bough or fallen tree. In contrast to the heat of the day, the temperature was comfortable with a refreshing breeze created by the speed of the craft. Encouraged by their success and fuelled by the excitement they took their speed up to twenty knots. As they changed over roles yet again they agreed that was the maximum safe limit of operation in those

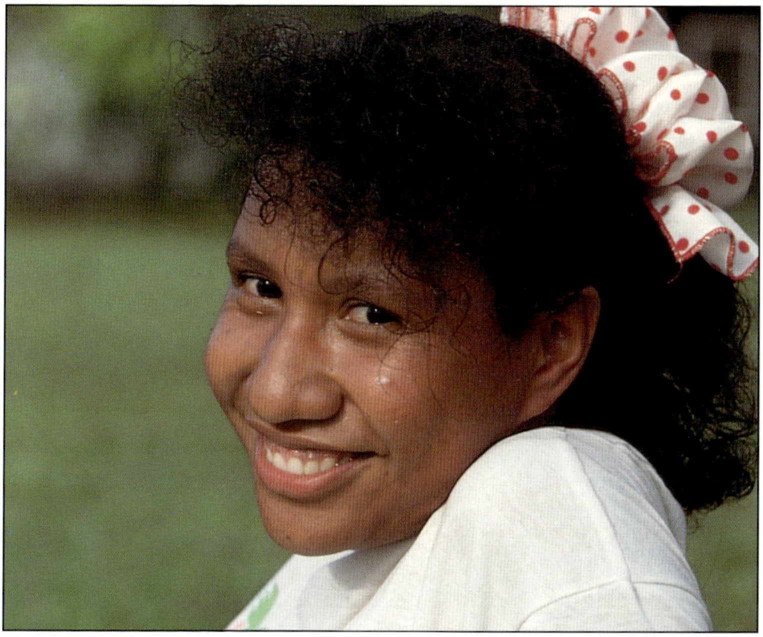

Above: Kila - first year nursing student
Below: Gogodala smiles

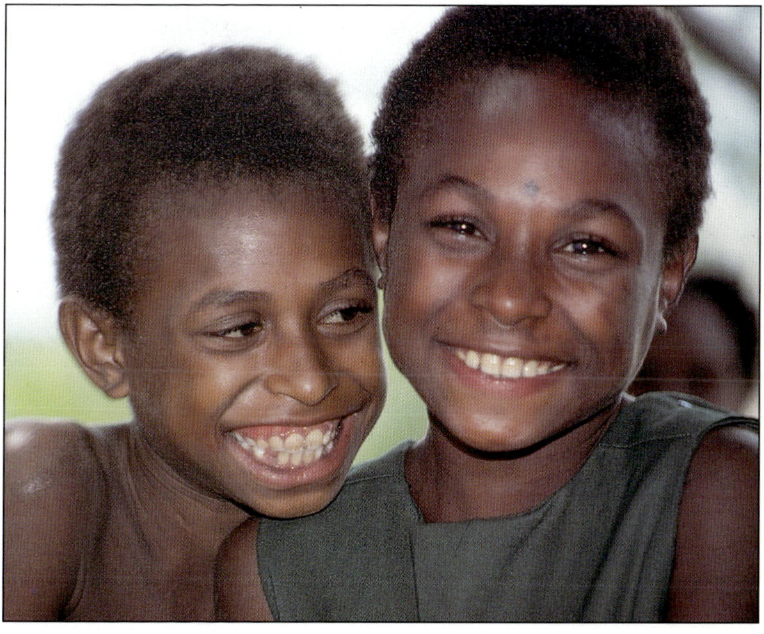

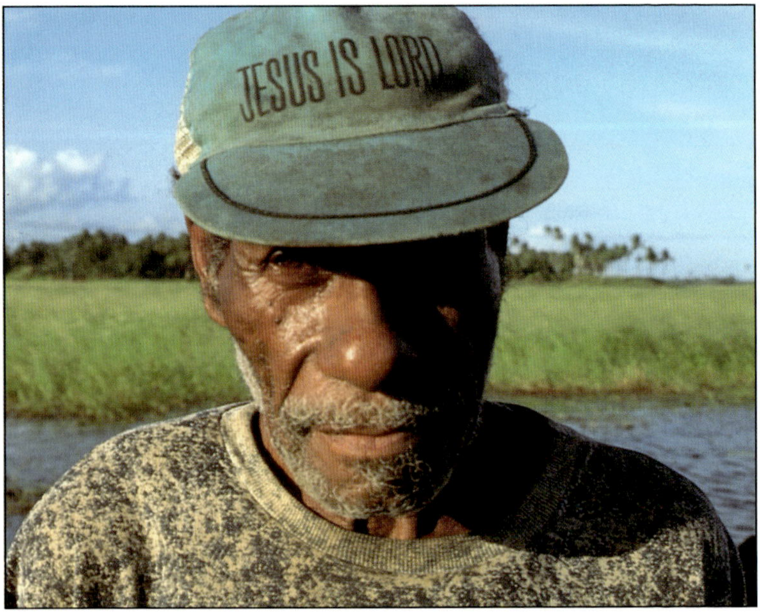

Above: A Gogodala Christian - fifty years of mission
Below: A do-it-yourself canoe
Right: Fly River delta village

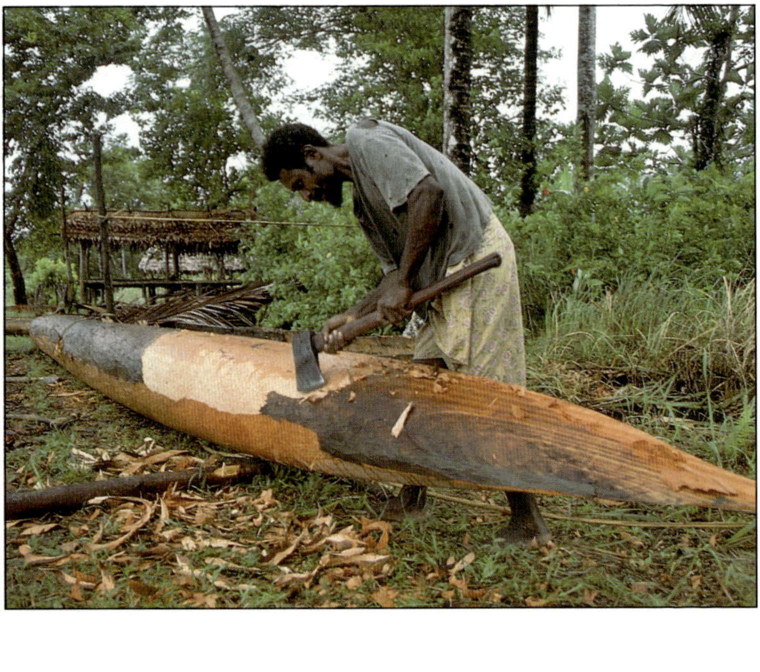

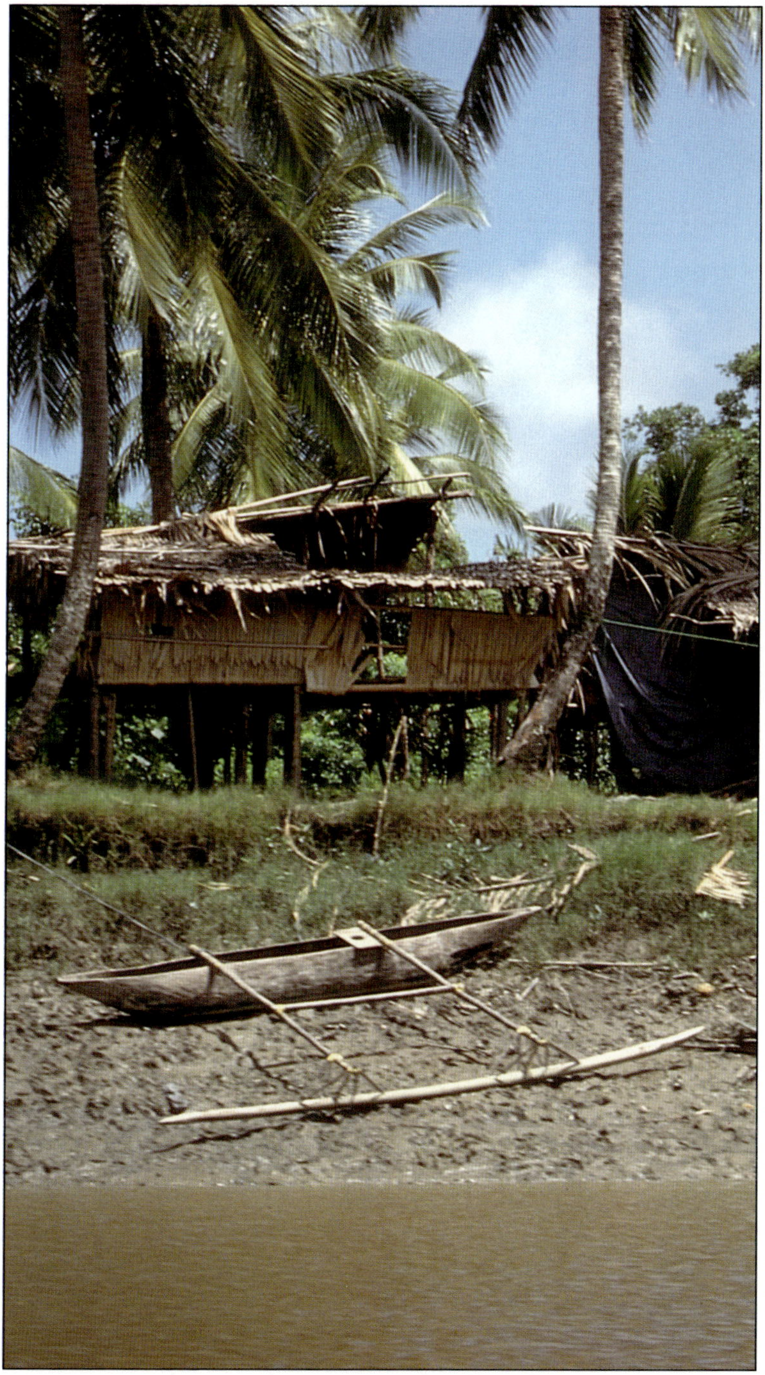

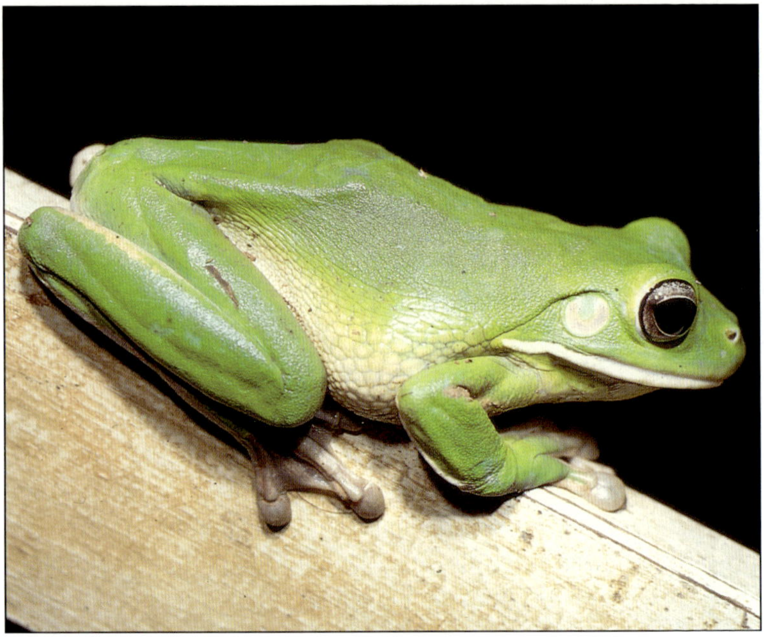

Above: High in the rafters
Below: Nature wears a beautiful cloak
Right: The enemy

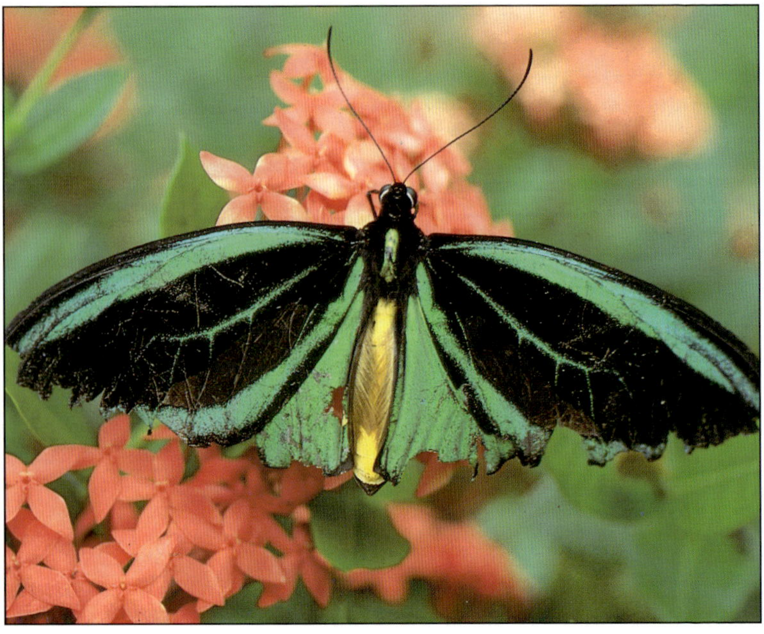

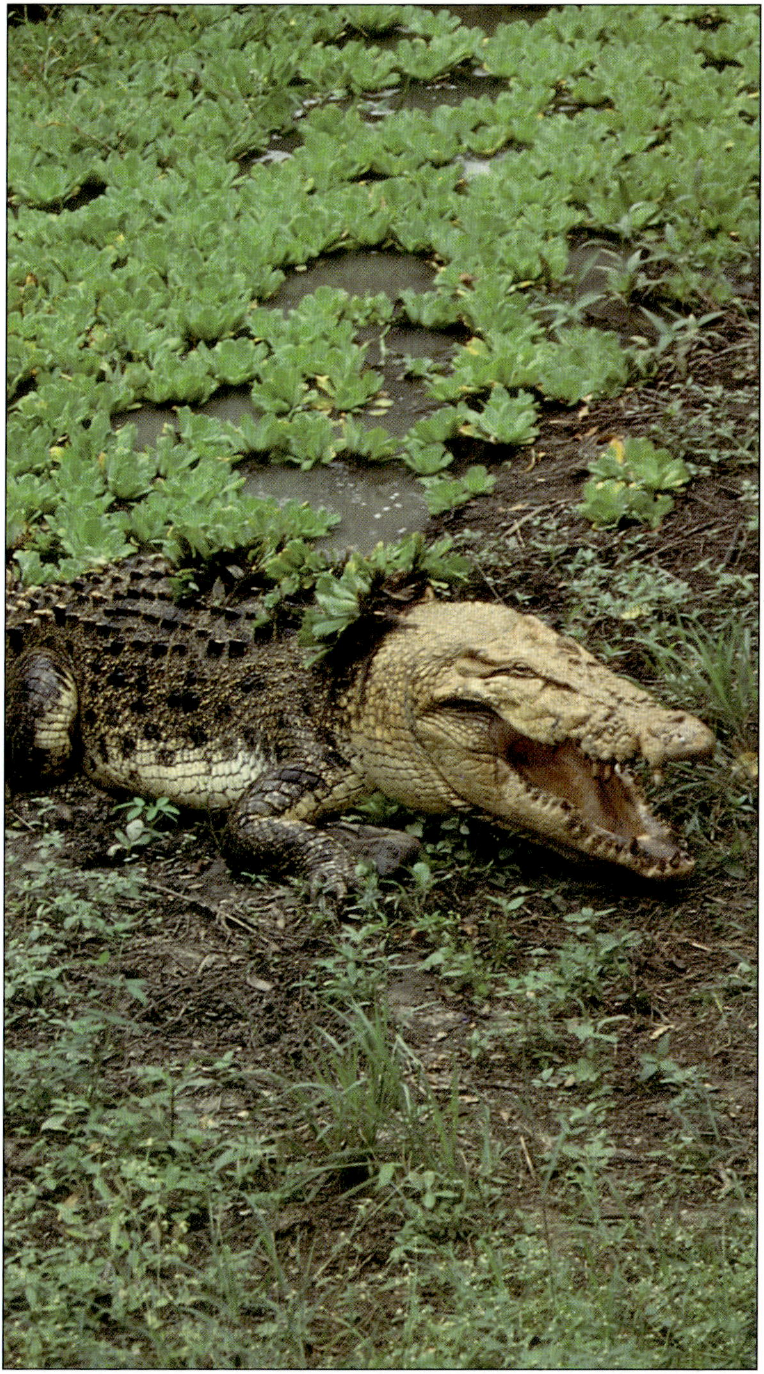

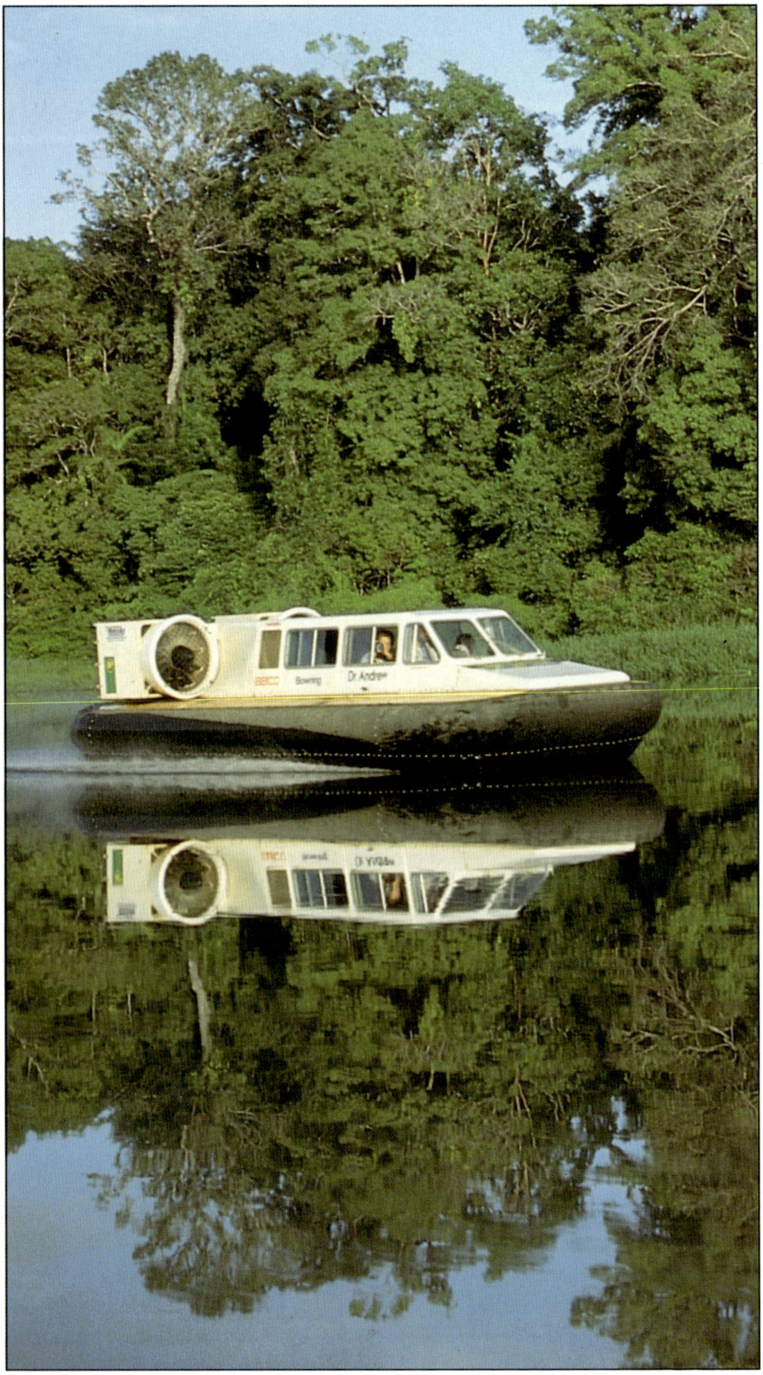

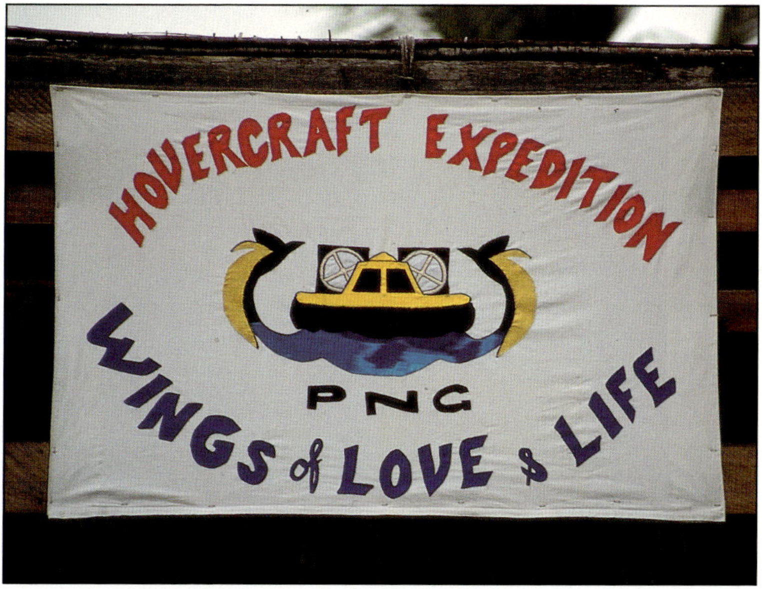

Left: Down the Bamu River at speed
Above: Hoverdoctor flag
Below: Wet fingers repairs downriver
Overpage: The lagoon

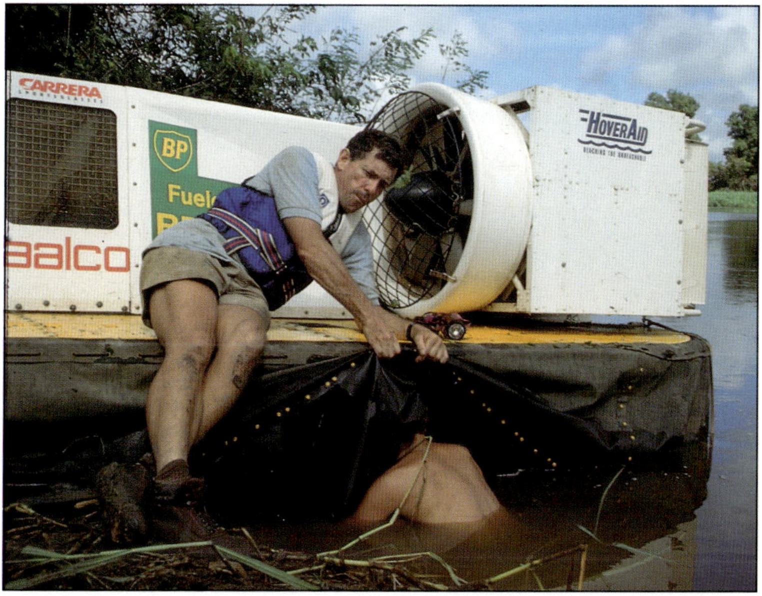

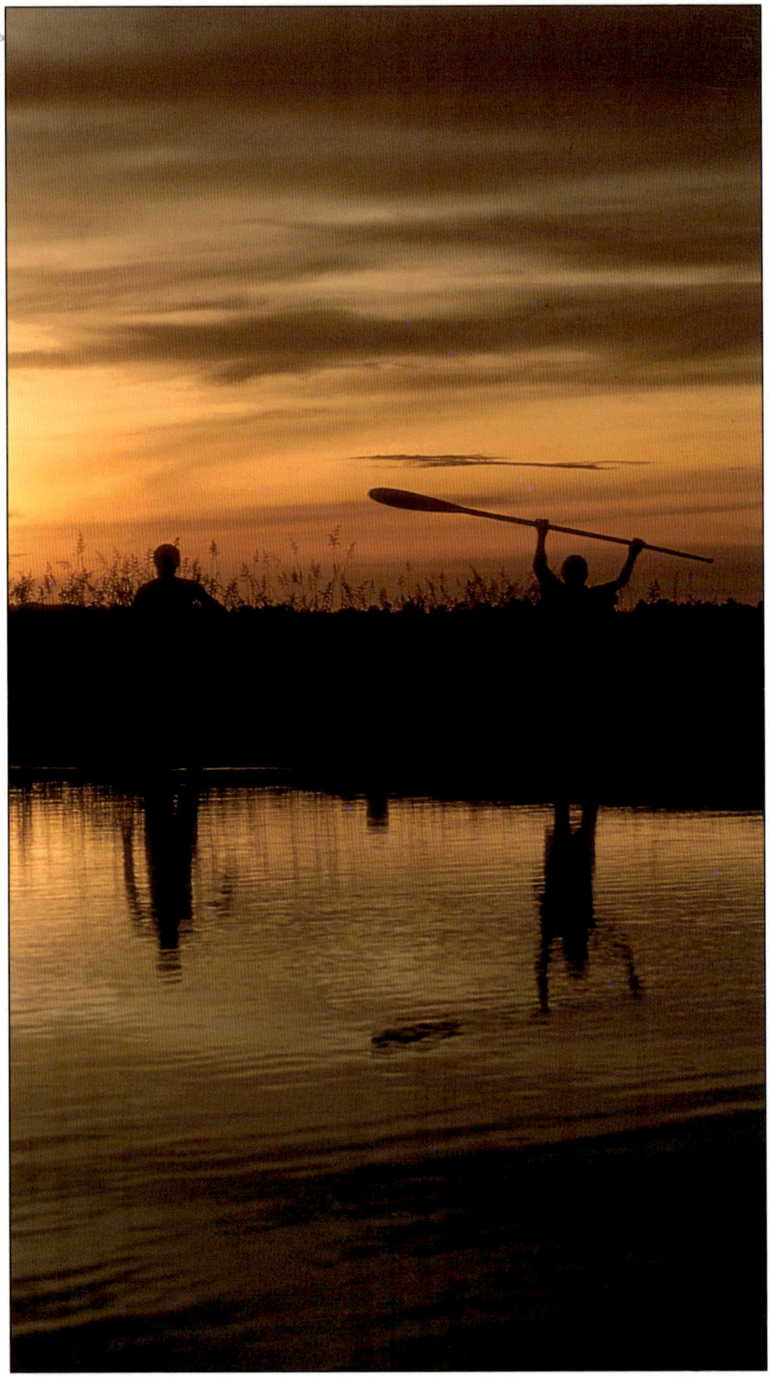

conditions with the light available.

Dropping speed as they entered the lagoon, they decided not to attempt to take the straight-line hovercraft track through the grass. That needed full power to overcome the resistance of the tall grasses and there would be the risk of losing the narrow channel that had been carved. Obstacles would also be more difficult to pick out. Instead, they followed the well-defined twisting channel. The torchlights on Mission Point were a welcome sight as they neared home. Gordon and Brian, alerted by radio from Saiwasi, were there to welcome them. Elated, the 'night riders' beached 402 in the usual spot. They had proved that the hovercraft could operate safely at night and at a speed much higher than anything else on the river. The hover ambulance was starting to show its potential.

To attempt a trial night-time run with only fit and healthy team members aboard is one thing; before it could be justified with a patient aboard more operational experience would be needed unless there was a real emergency. A possible one had confronted Graham Zerk as he held an impromptu outpatients' clinic at Mapodo. Never one to remain idle, Graham was making good use of his time while waiting for 402 to return from Balimo. That was when the severe prostate case was found. The man was in obvious pain from the bladder restriction and needed surgery. Graham decided he should be sent by hovercraft to Balimo as soon as it returned.

The hovercraft was delayed, however, and it was nearly dark by the time 402 arrived. Dr Zerk was faced with a difficult choice; either a night-time journey with a patient in pain and needing surgery or some means of relieving the condition temporarily, allowing a transfer in daylight. Graham decided to give the man some temporary relief, as the condition was not life-threatening. The Mapodo health sub-centre did not have the right tubing, so improvising with a length of oxygen tubing he drained off a litre of fluid from the patient. Much relieved, the man was settled in the health centre ward overnight and told he would be transferred the next day.

By seven o'clock the next morning the patient had disappeared. The man knew he had not been cured, but feeling much better, he had walked out. The inherent fear of surgery is very strong and often results in patients refusing to take advantage of the skills available to them. There was no alternative but to allow the hovercraft to return to Balimo without him.

Since the Moresby launch we had been referring to the hovercraft more by their names than their numbers. In the final preparations for the publicity launch Gordon had been able to put into effect the decision taken before we left the UK by placing his late mother's name on 402. Shortly before the expedition party left Britain Mrs Goodman had fallen ill and died and Gordon's father had generously supported the expedition in her memory. So, the second craft was named the *Jean Goodman*.

When 402 — the *Jean Goodman* — arrived at the hover-garage there was already plenty of activity as 401 — *Dr Andrew* — was being prepared for the exploratory probe next day down the Kenewa Creek. The outline maps of the area showed a series of creeks extending southwards towards the Fly, from the base of the huge U-shaped bend in the Aramia between Mapodo and Saiwasi. At that point the Aramia is nineteen miles (thirty kilometres) or so from the north bank of the Fly. The creeks extend for at least half that distance, petering out into swampy land. If the maps were accurate it was a possible way through to the Fly, potentially much shorter than the Bamu route and worth checking. The first hazard would be whether the entry creek from the Aramia itself was passable for hovercraft. That was to be checked by Graham Zerk and the film crew and a message passed back to Balimo. If it looked likely, both the *Jean Goodman* and the *Dr Andrew* would be used to explore the extent of navigable water and land in an attempt to reach the Fly.

Failing that, for whatever reason, the plan was to reach the Fly via the Bamu and Duro rivers and the Tirere Passage. Fuel had already been placed at Mapodo in preparation, but if the Kenewa Creek proved impassable, more might be needed from Emeti for the longer route. On its arrival preparation switched to RR 402 (*Jean Goodman*) so it too would be fully checked over, fuelled and provisioned ready for an early start the next morning. Later both craft were taken round to Mission Point and beached there, much to the excitement of the local children. By that time a call had already been received from Graham Zerk giving the thumbs down to Kenewa Creek. The hovercraft would be able to travel only a short way down it. The longer route would be the objective. In the course of that, it should be possible to call at Sisiama on Aramia Island in the mouth of the Bamu and visit Father Ronald Beauline, a French Canadian Roman Catholic priest based there.

He had appeared in the service one Sunday morning at the English-Speaking Church. Short, muscular and stocky, bronzed and wearing a chunky gold chain and cross easily visible in the widely opened neck of his short-sleeved shirt, he was anything but the conventional picture of a priest. Clearly at ease in the service despite the absence of any formal liturgy, he took the opportunity to introduce himself and explain the reason for his visit to Balimo. Father Ron, as he was readily called by all, was a lively, voluble character with a wonderful fund of stories with which he kept us entertained as he shared lunch at our invitation. Savage crocodiles, huge sharks with gaping jaws and high tidal bores all featured in his exciting tales, some inevitably with tragic endings.

At midnight on the Saturday, Father Ron had left Sisiama for Balimo in his launch. Starting off with only the light of a temporary spot lamp, he had motored along the rivers through the dark and on after dawn, up the Bamu and the Aramia arriving at the Balimo Health Centre after a seven-hour journey. With him were a pregnant woman and two of her family. The pregnancy was well advanced and seemed to be a potentially dangerous reverse presentation. Fearing a difficult delivery, Father Ron had thought he could delay departure no longer and was not at all confident that they would be able to reach Balimo in time. 'Calves I can cope with, but thees ... ' he said with a Gallic shrug. His fears were unfounded and the skills acquired over a number of years helping with calving on the family farm were not put to the ultimate test. All was well and the woman was delivered safely of a healthy baby later that day without undue complications. Some weeks earlier we had supplied Father Ron with some diesel fuel for his return journey and some to store for us as an emergency reserve at Sisiama. Now, while en route to the Fly there was an ideal opportunity to pay Father Ron a visit at Sisiama.

The two hovercraft left before seven, quickly getting over hump and making a splendid sight powering away in line through the grass-filled lagoon in the early morning sun. Steve, Amanda and Ben were in the *Andrew* while the *Jean* carried Graeme, Gordon and Chris Powell, the film crew producer. Only seven members were left at base now and they had a distinct feeling of anti-climax as they watched the craft disappear around the distant headland on their journey out beyond the lagoon.

The journey was uneventful as far as the fuel stop at Emeti. Graham Zerk and the rest of the film crew, with the dinghy, had linked up on the way through Mapodo and Saiwasi where there had been a pause for filming. By early afternoon the small flotilla of craft was ready to head down the Bamu which flows in a general south-easterly direction to the sea. A strong wind blew directly against the craft, creating very choppy water in the wide open expanse of the Bamu, which in places is more than one and three-quarter miles (three kilometres) across. These were not ideal conditions for small hovercraft and progress in the open water was painfully slow. Tackling the force of the wind head-on in open water proved not to be the best technique but it was a while before the right method was found.

The Bamu starts to widen and divide more than thirty miles (fifty kilometres) before it flows into the Gulf of Papua. Three large islands, Aramia, Damera and Naviu divide up the flow, separating it into three large rivers. One, the Bamu itself, runs down the north-eastern flank of Aramia Island.

By late afternoon the craft were still only part way along the shore of Aramia Island and still some distance from Sisiama, which lies on the southern end of the island, so it was decided to camp on the island overnight before continuing. The craft were beached and a fire started for the evening meal beneath a starlit sky. The hovercraft were used for sleeping, each covered by Jenny Smith's purpose-made large mosquito nets. Chris Powell decided he preferred to use a nearby empty fishing hut but managed to fall through the split palm floor, although without serious mishap. From Father Ron they knew that large aggressive crocodiles frequented the area but, despite that, everyone managed to have a good night's rest. By morning the hovercraft, beached the previous night, were gently swaying on the high tide. In the calm of the early morning they made good progress and were soon running up the creek approaching Sisiama village.

Sisiama, a village of about 200 people, lies on a huge mud flat, which is totally covered by the tide at least once a month. At low tide the mud seems to stretch forever, and there are many areas where it is easy to sink. There were about twenty houses in the village, all built on high stilts well above the mud. We had heard graphic descriptions of the conditions from Father Ron while he was at Balimo. As he came out to greet the unaccustomed visitors he managed to give a practical demonstration by sinking up to his waist in the mud. Despite the appalling conditions he had been at Sisiama for many years, caring for the villagers with the help of two Filipino nuns. A compo breakfast was shared and some interviews filmed in this unusual spot before the next leg of the journey began. The route lay south from Aramia Island down the Duro River, one of the three strands of the Bamu, between the tip of Aramia Island to the west and Naviu Island to the east, heading for the Tirere Passage. The Passage runs due south directly into the Fly estuary.

The *Jean Goodman* and the *Dr Andrew* headed south down the west shore of Naviu Island, leaving Ben, Amanda and two of the film crew with the dinghy at Sisiama. A strong south-easterly was blowing across the water again, but a new technique had been identified. By keeping in shallow water over the edge of the mud flats, the hovercraft could take advantage of the shielding effect of the jungle growth. The sudden shoaling of the water did not hinder the two craft, which skimmed easily on their air cushions over water or land. Making good speed, they progressed along the

Naviu shoreline until well beyond the mouth of the Tirere Passage on the opposite side of the Duro River. The hovercraft then swung on to a westerly course, heading for the mouth of the Tirere Passage, riding the waves well above hump speed across one and three-quarter miles (three kilometres) of open water with the full advantage of a strong tailwind.

The calm of the Tirere Passage was a startling contrast. As they passed villages on the banks, children waved and yelled. The hovercraft might as well have come from outer space as far as they were concerned; they had never seen anything like them before. The rest of the villagers had a different and more aggressive attitude, fearing for the safety of their nets. These were poor people living at subsistence level, very much dependent on fishing for their survival. Knowing only propeller-driven craft, they were convinced that if the hovercraft went over their nets they would be ripped apart. They had no way of knowing that only the edges of the rubber skirt make contact with the surface as a hovercraft skims over the water.

As the two craft neared the end of the four-mile (six kilometre) passage the water had shoaled until it was only inches deep, impassable for boats with outboards or even canoes. In these conditions, the hovercraft is supreme. With a great sense of elation and thanksgiving the crews paused in the craft on a huge mud flat. The Fly River had been reached, at 00.45 hrs GMT on 29 April 1993.

The south-western side of the massive delta lay more than thirty-seven miles (sixty-odd kilometres) away entirely out of sight. The nearest land was just over six miles (ten kilometres) distant, the north bank of one of the many large islands that make up the delta system. Seeing a lone figure on a mud bank, they drove over and parked the craft near him. To their amazement, in this sparsely populated area so far from Balimo, he turned out to be a former patient of Dr Tucker. Five years before, Graham Tucker had operated on him with Graham Zerk acting as anaesthetist. Greetings were exchanged and soon, twenty or more fishermen appeared from nowhere and gathered around watching with great interest while some finger ties torn off in the waves were replaced. The occasion was recorded on film before they left to return via the Tirere Passage.

As they passed the impoverished villages on the way back, the greetings were quite different, with delighted waves replacing the earlier aggression. No doubt there had been a frantic scramble to check the precious fishing nets after the first passage. The villagers would have been astonished to find them intact and now they were only too ready to treat this strange craft and those who came in it in a friendly way. That is important for the future; the expedition has shown that the hovercraft can be relied on to reach out beyond the present range of the Balimo service into areas that previously could not be given any help. If ever the opportunity arises to extend the service, a friendly reception for the health care that the craft brings could be of great value in achieving good results.

The villages in the area are very needy; disease is rife and the health of the people is getting worse. It is not melodramatic to say that the tribes in the area are facing extinction unless health care can reach them before long. With proper fuel dumps on the way, the area could be reached from Balimo. The possibility is there but not the resources. In 1992, the second year of a three-year contract, the government grant to the health centre was cut by almost one-third. As a result, it struggles to cope with its present workload. Until resources are increased nothing more can be done. If they are not increased in the future, even the present work is threatened. The Minister for Health's acknowledgment of the good work that is done is appreciated, but alone it does not help those who still lack the opportunity of being treated when they are sick. A partnership with the voluntary agencies is an excellent way of making good use of scarce government resources, but the partnership needs to be balanced, not lopsided. The hovercraft have provided the means of reaching out beyond the range of the present service but taking advantage of that will be impossible without the appropriate level of medical backup . For the people in these needy villages a lot depends on this issue.

Sisiama was visited on the return journey, surplus stores left with Father Ron and fuel taken on board for the trip home. With a tailwind and the mudflat-hopping technique, great progress was made up the Bamu, speeds of over thirty knots being recorded at times. The degree of change in the river systems was considerable (assuming the accuracy of the 1965 maps). Over one stretch of river the GPS equipment showed the hovercraft to be more than a mile (about one and a half kilometres) inland. The changes result from a combination of silting up and jungle decay. As a consequence, part-submerged trees dot the shallow water and a very sharp watch must be kept for these major hazards that can spell sudden death to a hovercraft. Steve was steering adroitly between two of these obstacles when all too late it was realised that the two were one, both being ends of a very large tree trunk. The crew shouted warnings and braced themselves for the impact, but it never came. They were through without damage; what a relief.

The two craft were running close together at times. That gave Steve a chance to observe the way the *Jean* was sitting on the water. The lower part of the skirt, the fingers, should have been almost fully visible but only about one-third was showing; the rest was in the water. This was another observation that made sense later.

Without further incident, Mapodo was reached, and the long-suffering missionaries there and at Saiwasi divided the travellers between them once more for another overnight stop. With only the Mapodo-to-Balimo stretch to cover the next day, there was plenty of time on the return journey for the film crew to get lots of footage of the two hovercraft travelling up and down the river and calling at the riverside villages. There was certainly plenty of interest and co-operation from the inhabitants. One little boy became so excited, bouncing up and down on the end of a log, that he fell in the river. The whole trip was rounded off on the group's return to Balimo by the graduation ceremony for the nurses and the open air 'feast' which followed, Brian remarking that there was enough food to satisfy even Ben's gargantuan appetite! It seemed a very fitting celebration after the excitement of the Fly adventure.

There had been careful preparations around Mission Point in readiness for the formal handover of the two hovercraft on Wednesday 5 May. There was to be a ceremony attended by the Minister for Health, Francis Koinmanrea, and the British High Commissioner, John Guy. The training of the four nationals had been continuing and they had now reached a good standard of proficiency both in driving and maintenance of the craft. Ilaba and Dekame had made such good progress that Ilaba had been able to take part in training Sebia and Olo who had previously had fewer opportunities for training than the others. It was intended that on 5 May all the driving would be done by Ilaba and Dekame.

The Monday started quietly, with the intention of thoroughly cleaning the two craft for the big occasion. That was soon interrupted when a radio call came through from Tim Schlatter at

Saiwasi. A twenty-five-year-old man, Kubili, had been brought to him after having been bitten on the leg by a deadly Papuan death adder. Tim had applied a bandage to the leg and was about to take Kubili to the Mapodo health sub-centre. As the sub-centre had no antivenene, it was essential for a doctor to get to Mapodo with it in the shortest possible time. A two-and-a-half-hour journey by outboard canoe would almost certainly be too late.

Graham Zerk was alerted at the hospital. Collecting his kit and the essential antivenene, he was driven to Mission Point where the *Jean Goodman* was being prepared. With Dekame driving, they made a record dash of just over an hour to Mapodo. Kubili was in a bad way, unable to swallow or open his eyes, and barely able to breathe. Gradually, over the prescribed period of half an hour, Graham Zerk carefully administered the antivenene serum. For a further hour he monitored Kubili's progress to ensure there were no adverse reactions. He also managed to see a few other patients. Within two hours Kubili was well on the way to recovery, able to swallow and even talk. Had there been a delay in getting the right treatment, he would certainly have died.

It made a moving contrast to the incident witnessed by Mike Cole on his reconnaissance visit. Then, a young boy, Maidame Kukupi, had been brought to Balimo after being bitten by a poisonous snake. There had been a delay in getting him to the hospital for treatment and he had died. In Kubili's case the hovercraft had made the difference we had been striving for, and it more than justified all our effort. There was now scope for many such timely interventions by hovercraft in the years to come. It was not Kubili's first narrow escape, we learned later. Only a year before he had been bitten on the backside by a crocodile and lived to tell the tale. Perhaps he would curb his adventuring a little.

We had been warned not to take chances; we had seen the snakes for ourselves. While they were not numerous, there were also crocodiles around the area and hearing of Kubili's earlier experience was a reminder. These were not the larger estuarine variety of crocodile, such as Father Ron had told us about. Nevertheless, being up to twelve feet (about four metres) in length they posed a considerable threat if they chose to try and add a human to their diet. Graham Tucker had made the point about their presence in and around the lagoon by his account of an unfortunate woman who had been fishing. Out on the lagoon she had reverted to traditional dress and was clad only in a wrapa-round skirt. Leaning over the side of her canoe tending her net she had been seized by a crocodile and had an 'instant mastectomy' as Graham had put it. He had the job of repairing the damaged breast as best he could.

Graham Zerk's drama was not over for the day after treating Kubili. Later that evening he was routinely attending the delivery of a baby, supervising the maternity sister. The delivery was straightforward but when born, the baby's airways were filled with mucus. This happens rarely and the sister was not qualified to handle the situation. The child's airways had to be aspirated and then drained four times by the doctor before the danger had passed.

With our Westernised expectation of a medical service, it is easy to overlook the workload of these dedicated doctors. Had it not been for Graham Zerk's involvement with the hovercraft project, the whole workload would have fallen on Graham Tucker alone. His own case load was already considerable, in addition to being administrator of the Balimo Health Centre. The occasional help of colleagues such as Drs Ramsay and Zerk was not only welcome to ease the load briefly, but essential in giving a much-needed respite from time to time.

Dr Ray Pinniger and I were able to look at the provision of medical services in another part of PNG. The Ok Tedi Mining Co had flown us to Tabubil to see the company-run hospital there. The company was interested in the hovercraft project and was considering whether to give some financial help from the Fly River Trust which the company had set up. The huge copper mine, the fifth largest in the world, is situated in the mountains of Papua New Guinea above the town of Tabubil, only eleven miles (eighteen kilometres) from the border with Irian Jaya, the Indonesian part of the New Guinea island. The mine is on the Ok Tedi, a tributary of the Fly, and the Trust had been set up to finance projects for the benefit of the people living along the length of the Fly River, the main transport route for mine's exports. Unfortunately it was decided that the Trust could not give financial help, but the company did give some assistance by flying members of the team from Balimo to Port Moresby at the conclusion of the project.

The Tabubil Health Centre is a model of its kind. Dr Paul Spicer showed us around with justifiable pride. Every facility is available in the hospital and the standard of the equipment is excellent. There is also a medical service for the mining company employees. The contrast with the Balimo Hospital is stark. Each receives a similar level of grant from the government but, whereas the 120-bed hospital at Balimo has to function on little more than the government grant, the twenty-bed Tabubil Health Centre funded by the mining company has a budget more than twice the amount of the grant. The standard of medical care being provided from Tabubil is excellent, as it is at Balimo, but the level of investment in equipment and the standards of finish in wards and treatment areas is lavish by comparison.

Dr Spicer is the chief medical officer at Tabubil and has the support of another doctor. He carries the responsibility for the service provided by the hospital which serves the mining town of Tabubil and some of the mountain settlements around the area. That represents a considerable workload, but the centre has a staffing level similar to that of the much larger hospital at Balimo. The malaria and filariasis control programme operated in the area, and any emergency visits are able to call on company resources for the use of a helicopter. Some of the industrial accidents that occur, covered by the company medical service, can even be referred to specialist services in large Australian hospitals. Yet the hospital at Balimo with its complement of one doctor, with occasional extra help and modest facilities, serves the whole of the Western Fly Province with a population of over 100,000 people. The addition of the hovercraft service will help make better use of its modest resources, but the imbalance in financing will still be great.

Our involvement in the project to aid the hospital at Balimo had taught us that the Gogodala are a quiet, gentle people long influenced by the teaching of the missionaries who had first settled at Balimo in 1931. A high proportion of the people were at least nominally Christian and church attendance was thought to be as high as eighty per cent. Changes were coming about, however, as the influences of the wider world were felt. They were visible in other ways too. In a society where formerly all waste products were organic and therefore biodegradable the litter of modern packaging could be seen around Balimo, particularly soft drink cans and bottles. The very frequently seen outboard motors were further evidence of outside influences. We were conscious of being instruments for change, too. The hovercraft we had brought would have their effect and in some way speed up change. It seems very difficult to introduce only beneficial change or to control the direction or pace once the process has started. Elsewhere in PNG the effects are more pronounced than in Balimo. That was clear from my own visits to Moresby and Tabubil and, as Sarah and Aileen found out, in Hagen in the Highlands also.

Sarah and Aileen had decided to pay a visit to Hagen as they left Balimo. As they were driven from the airstrip by their hostess, they were told that the bridge they were crossing was often ambushed. No sooner had they settled into the house where they were to stay than they saw smoke coming from nearby houses that had been set on fire in local tribal fighting. The mission hospital that had treated some wounded from one tribe has also been threatened with fire by the opposing tribe. Shots were heard and men started running around with guns. This was worrying enough in itself, but more so when Sarah and Aileen were told that the tribespeople did not know how to use the guns properly.

Tribal war is part of the cultural fabric of PNG, especially in the Highlands. There, where the pressure on land has been more severe than in the Fly and other districts, war between tribes is common and is rooted in the past. Traditionally it has been a means of settling disputes. It still occurs largely because the modern methods for conflict resolution are not seen to be effective. To a significant extent, the efforts of the colonial powers to end tribal warfare in the coastal areas were successful; often punitive expeditions were used. Those methods are not open to the authorities today and no successful method of stamping out the wars in the Highlands has been found. This presents the police with a huge problem, according to a former police commissioner.

Until the 1970s, only traditional weapons — bows and arrows, spears and clubs — were used by the tribes. Then guns started to appear. Many are homemade and some blow up in the hands of the users. The appearance of guns seems also to have extended the range of disputes that trigger wars; often they are petty.

There are no simple solutions to such flare-ups. In the Western Province and in the Aramia River area in particular, the people live at peace, free of most of the less desirable features of change that have adversely affected many of their countrymen. It is a fragile balance that needs to be nurtured with care and sensitivity. Yet in doing that it would be wrong, in my view, to stand aside from opportunities to relieve suffering or save life.

12

Over and Out

The project was now entering its final phase. Soon the formal handover ceremony would take place. The team was decreasing in size as members came to the end of the time they were able to spend on the project. The performance of the two hovercraft had been improved considerably and they were running reliably, but the engineers hoped to produce yet more power. Exploratory trips west of the operational area still had to be made, to identify better and shorter routes through the grass swamp lagoon areas upriver in contrast to the 'open water' runs downriver to the east and through to the Fly. The medical patrols spent much of their time in the western areas and any saving the hovercraft team could identify would be of great value in making better use of the medical staff.

Handover day was to be a big local event and a great deal of effort was being put into the preparation by the Gogodala people. Mission Point had been transformed by a team of thirty or more of the local pastors, wielding their long grass knives. The term 'pastor' in the Fly area carries a different meaning from that in the UK. There it usually implies the responsibility for the leadership of a church, and overseeing the spiritual welfare of the church membership. In the Fly area and elsewhere in Papua New Guinea 'pastor' may mean that, but it generally implies a wider role in the community. The pastors have all been to Bible College for varying periods and so their education has progressed beyond the normal schooling available to most people, so they are expected to provide more general leadership within the community. A church may then have a number of pastors in its congregation.

In the preparations for the ceremony, the pastors were certainly leading by example. Within a day, they had cut down the long grass over the two high spits of land that jutted out from Mission Point and formed a viewpoint overlooking the lagoon. Working hard in the open sun, they did not seem to need the frequent intake of liquid that we had found essential. They worked on an informal rota. A number were always standing around in the light shade of the coconut palms and periodically a man would step forward to replace one of those at work, who would then take a break in the shade. In this way the work proceeded continuously, with some always refreshed and ready to carry on.

Lunch break in the hottest part of the day did not involve lying around; instead, it was spent harvesting green coconuts. Several of the younger men shinned barefoot up the tall slender palm trunks to the cluster of large fronds at the top. With the soles of their feet angled on either side of the trunk and hands gripping the trunk at a higher level, they moved up the tree in a series of smooth movements until they disappeared out of sight among the palm fronds. There, in the angle of the fronds and the trunk were the clusters of green fruits. Hacking with machetes or simply pushing with their feet, the men dislodged the nuts. Falling from their high perch, the nuts hit the ground with force. A few times I had woken in the night to the loud crash of a coconut bouncing off the roof after being dislodged by the wind.

We were told that the young coconut milk was the best and were given the opportunity to sample it. It was hard to associate the objects on the ground with the brown hairy coconuts we buy in the UK. They were larger than the nuts familiar to us, green, not brown, smooth, not hairy. One of the pastors took his knife and with deft strokes hacked the top of the outer green casing into a pointed shape, revealing a white pithy layer below. With the point of his knife he cut out a hole in the top of the nut. Inside we could see the moist white fleshy layer and, swilling around in the centre, the sweet milk. It tasted refreshing, nature's original pure packaged soft drink.

Curious about the packaging I later cut into the green outer casing to investigate. It was surprisingly tough. Beneath the outer casing lay the brown fibrous layer of the husk, from which useful coconut matting is made. Finally came the familiar hairy shell housing the flesh and the milk. As a tribe of gatherers the Gogodala make much use of this naturally occurring food as a flavouring for sago. Several of the pastors were scraping out the flesh with a piece of the shell, possibly their only lunch. Others were loosening strands of the outer husks and tying two together, so forming a carrying handle ready to take the nuts home to the family later.

Grass cutting was not the only preparation for the big day. At Kimama, south across the lagoon from Balimo, much effort had gone into practising for a canoe race. This is very much part of Gogodala cultural tradition. The low-lying floodplain area is inundated with water for much of the year, making canoes the only practicable daily means of transport between the numerous grassy hillocks on which the individual family huts are built.

Ceremonial canoes are very elaborate in comparison with the workaday ones. Intricately carved with clan totems on the prow and sometimes on the stern, the racing canoes are often pigmented with further designs. The carvings or the paintings can take the form of a Gi, a devouring monster, swallowing a hornbill, a crocodile swallowing a cockatoo, or a pig swallowing a sea eagle. Each of the creatures, real or mythological, represents a clan totem or sub-totem.

The tribe has a complex social structure that often bemused us. It is divided several times over into a number of sub-clans each with its own totemic emblem, or *Gawa Tao* (see *Gogodala, Lagoon Dwellers of the Gulf* by A. I. Crawford published by Robert Brown & Associates, Bathurst, NSW, Australia). The design of the *Gawa Tao* is applied to all ceremonial paraphernalia and is sometimes painted on the bodies of the performers in the Maiyata, one of the two major rituals of the culture. Taking part in the canoe races involved not only physical work but also making and wearing the traditional body decorations of pigment, leaves and chest bands with, topping it all, the *Diwa*, a woven grass conical hat. Much use is made of colourful croton leaves which are still grown for ceremonial purposes, although not on the scale of pre-Christian times.

As a result of the pastors' labours, Mission Point was looking fine on 5 May, the day of the handover ceremony. It was a beautiful morning and the team made an early start with breakfast at 6 am. Some were involved in the handover ceremony and the rest were going off with Pastor Sika, the official starter of the canoe race that was to take place on the Aramia beyond the lagoon entrance. As they went out through the lagoon they saw heavy traffic of canoes coming in the opposite direction full of eager people on their way to Balimo for the ceremony. Even the barge *MV Aramia* was in service, packed with an excited crowd from Kawito. There were three races for different-sized canoes with between eighteen and twenty-four crew paddling in each. With a common finishing line each category of canoe started at a different point on the river. It made a splendid sight to see the leaf-decorated crews dipping their painted bodies in unison as they thrust their long carved and decorated paddles into the water with powerful strokes, chanting as they did so.

At Balimo the official guests started to arrive at 9.30 am, having flown out from Port Moresby that morning. Principal guests were the PNG Minister for Health Francis Koinmanrea the British High Commissioner John Guy and the two Members of Parliament from the Middle Fly and the Western Province. They were collected from the airstrip with other guests, including Dr Paul Spicer from Tabubil, and driven to the Biula church close to the school in Balimo. There the hospital staff gave them a musical welcome as well as a dramatised version of the arrival of the first missionaries at Balimo in 1931 and the growth of the local work of the Evangelical Church of Papua New Guinea since then.

Refreshments followed at Jill Adams' house nearby at Mission Point, so leaving the guests well placed for the official arrival there of the *Jean Goodman* and the *Dr Andrew* driven by Dekame and Ilabe. Gordon and Graeme arrived in the *Jean* and Steve and Graham Zerk in the *Dr Andrew*. There was an official welcome from Gordon in front of a huge crowd and then the official guests and Paul Spicer went off across the lagoon in the *Jean* with Dekame and the two MPs in the *Dr Andrew* with Ilabe. On their return, speeches followed, including one in Gogodala by Graham Zerk. In his speech the minister praised the work of the health centre and said he was impressed with the work of the hospital and its facilities. He declared his intention to designate the Centre a 'district hospital', one of many he saw as a means of improving the health of the people of PNG. (It will be interesting to learn the effect of any such designation, as Balimo already carries out more work than the provincial hospital at Daru but does not get the same recognition, nor even the full amount of its agreed grant.)

The hospital and the school of nursing were toured by the official party. During the course of the tour the Health Minister visited Samson Zeipi, the younger brother of Environment and Conservation Minister Perry Zeipi, who was a patient in the hospital. The party then inspected the hover-garage and workshop built by the team. In front of the Council Chamber the Kini Cult Dance Group gave a demonstration of traditional dancing in full Gogodala decoration. Lunch was served to the party in the Biula church before the guests took their leave in mid-afternoon, by which time the hovercraft team were exhausted but exhilarated. The official ceremony was over, but there was still work to be done.

Ali was one focus of that work. It lies on the Aramia almost forty-four miles (seventy kilometres) north-west of Balimo, but very much further by water, at the limit of the present canoe range of the medical patrols. Gordon was concerned to find any ways of reducing the distance by using shortcuts the hovercraft could take. Originally he had been keen to see if there might be any feasible route from the Aramia at Ali through to the Fly, but an aerial reconnaissance had shown that would not be possible.

Fuel dumps along the route would be necessary because of the distance involved. Ideally four or five drums of diesel would have been dumped at Makapa. The best that could be done was to send up one of the hovercraft with the equivalent of one full drum of diesel and get as far as possible on that. Jonathan Allan and Michael Pinkess were given the task. The plan was to drive to Kawito and pick up fuel, at the same time dropping off Martin Healey for other tasks there. With the extra fuel on board they would go as far as Makapa where the diesel would be placed ready for the two hovercraft to use en route for Ali. That done, Martin was to be collected and the three were to return to Balimo before dark the same day. It all sounded quite feasible in theory.

After the *Dr Andrew* had been checked at base, the journey to Kawito was uneventful; it was now so familiar that it had become routine. Dropping off Martin, Jonathan and Michael filled up the fuel tanks and half filled two fuel drums, which they just managed to manhandle into the cabin, where they fitted snugly. With the full tanks, the extra fuel and themselves, the hovercraft had a fair payload. During the journey they explored some possible short cuts across the lagoons which Gordon had spotted from the air while on a recce flight with Paul, a national pilot who had replaced Bruce Turner at the Kawito MAF base.

On the way to Makapa Jonathan handed over the driving to Michael, who had had little opportunity to drive before. Conditions were not the best. A blustery wind made the water choppy and the weight of the extra fuel sloshing around in the two half-full drums made the craft difficult to handle. A sudden gust of wind dumped the craft heavily in the water for an instant, ripping out some finger ties on the nearside rear corner. The water tore at the loose skirt fingers, increasing the drag as the fabric flapped in the water, threatening yet more damage. But the river banks had grown in to the water's edge and there was nowhere they could get off the water. With no alternative, they had to press on until they reached Awaba where the hovercraft could be beached. By that time the damage was worse and it took an hour and a half to repair, lying on banana leaves on the muddy bank half under the skirt, watched all the time by a crowd of curious spectators.

Not long after the expedition stated off again, the entrance to a lagoon came in sight. According to the map it offered a significant short cut. Checking on the Global Positioning Equipment (GPS) they decided this was the right spot. At first the channel was wide and clearly defined, but soon it petered out and the expanse of the grass-covered lagoon confronted them. They stopped to take stock. The lagoon covered many square miles, stretching almost as far as the eye could see and bordered only in the distance by a fringe of trees. Tall grasses growing up through the water waved gracefully in the now-gentle breeze; in places tough-looking reeds offered a more substantial barrier. Patches of open water were carpeted with a burgundy-red moss punctuated by the widespread leaves of water lilies, their pink or white flowers wide open to the sun.

Taking a bearing from the map for the most likely exit on the northern side, they started on a straight line course. This was the terrain where the hovercraft really could show its unique qualities and they decided to put it to the test. With maximum thrust to prevent getting bogged down, Michael headed the craft into the grass. Forward visibility was limited and the adrenalin flowed as they pushed ahead. Jonathan had his work cut out as he tried to keep track of their progress on the GPS, guiding Michael on the right bearing and at the same time keeping an eye on his driving technique.

The reeds, looking much more formidable as the craft raced towards them, towered above the cabin roof. Without noticeable impact they ploughed into them, finding them not as densely packed as imagined and offering little resistance as they were pushed flat to the water. After a minute of blind progress and with reeds still ahead, doubts crept in as to the wisdom of their action. A dull thud on the underside of the craft indicated that they had skimmed down the side of a waterlogged tree trunk low in the water. Entering a patch of clear water, they stopped to check on progress. Jonathan had to climb on the roof of the cabin to get a view. There, only ten feet (three metres) to their right was a fast-flowing open channel. Travelling blindly, they had arrived almost exactly at the exit from the lagoon. What a duo! Boosted by self-congratulation they drove the craft out through the reeds into the channel, through a narrow cut in the red clay bank, and then they popped like a cork out of a bottle onto the main river itself, the thrust fans shredding their way through the leaves of an overhanging tree.

Makapa lay further upriver on the edge of another large lagoon. A channel through tall reeds linked it to the river. Passing along the channel they saw people waving to them from the bank. This lagoon was different; instead of the now-familiar tall grass, there was a covering of short grassy weed floating on the surface waiting to tangle around the propeller of any outboard motor unwisely driven into it. It looked like a huge flat bowling green, broken up in places by narrow clear water channels. *Jean* skimmed swiftly over the surface, taking a slalom course around the tall bamboo poles that marked the ends of fishing nets staked in the water.

Near the village on the edge of the lagoon, the grass changed to the tall familiar type. Suddenly, the craft came to a stop. With a groan, Jonathan recognised from earlier experience what had happened: the craft was sitting on a mat of grass over solid ground, not water. Lift pressure was being lost as the packed-down grass prevented the skirt from making a seal with either solid earth or water. There was only one solution. Cutting the engine they climbed over the side and started pulling the grass out from under the edges of the skirt. It was laborious work in the blazing sun and hard on the hands, too, as the coarse grass cut into their skin.

After about half an hour they had had enough, and they started up the hovercraft in the hope it might be possible to get away. Michael gave it maximum thrust and juggled all the controls to try to get the craft off the grass. Jonathan pushed, pulled and jumped up and down on the nose of the craft until he was exhausted. Nothing happened until, after a pause and with a prayer of desperation, they tried once more. Painfully slowly, the craft edged forward. Standing on the nose of the craft Jonathan guided Michael towards the main channel.

With success in sight and only fifteen feet (five metres) short of the open water, they ground to a halt again. Wearily they set to work once more, heaving out the grass. Soon they became aware of a canoe coming down the channel towards them. Six men landed and approached them carrying long knives. Raising his hand, the leading man said, 'We are with the Lord.' With relief, Jonathan blurted out, 'Thank goodness for that, so are we!' as he took the proffered hand. Two of the men introduced themselves as pastors of the church in Makapa. In no time at all, the gang had slashed a clear swathe between the craft and the main channel.

Owami, one of the pastors, came on board to guide them to the village. At the water's edge stood a large crowd of villagers. Several of the men readily helped to unload the two barrels and, leaving the fuel in Owami's care, they started off on a different route out of the lagoon to avoid running aground again.

It was no simple matter to find the channel back to the river. They saw women fishing in the middle of the lagoon and drew alongside to ask for help. Ever the gentleman, Michael enquired in his careful English, 'Excuse me, I'm awfully sorry to trouble you, but could you tell me the way to Balimo, please?' Giggles and embarrassed laughter were the only response. Recovering themselves the women pointed out a channel and told them to turn left on reaching the river. As the hovercraft moved off, Michael and Jonathan themselves collapsed in laughter at the sheer absurdity of their Englishness on a remote PNG lagoon.

A sense of the surreal continued as they neared the river. Their way was blocked by a man in a canoe who was beckoning to them. As they drew alongside he handed up an envelope. 'Will you post this for me, please?' he said passing it over with a 50-toea coin. 'Yes, of course,' they managed to reply in astonishment. What else might they encounter in this area that was once populated by head hunters?

By now the 'hovering fuel-tanker' was way behind schedule. At the entrance to the short cut across the lagoon west of Awaba, Jonathan and Michael conferred. Little more than half an hour of daylight was left and the thought of navigating across the lagoon in failing light did not appeal, much less the possibility of getting stuck in the dark. But with time against them, they decided to take the risk as they had the GPS to guide them. On the way out they had recorded in the GPS memory the various 'waymark' points and could replay them in reverse for the return journey.

Initially they made good progress, following visually what they thought to be a straight line route towards the exit point. But almost becoming bogged down in dense grass alerted them that somewhere they must have gone astray. The GPS showed they had gone too far into the lagoon and so missed the exit channel. In very poor light they retraced their route. Then, by constantly cross-referencing their GPS position to the terrain shown on the map, they found the channel again and with relief followed it to the river. It was now almost dark, so they stopped and waited a little time for their night vision to improve. Jonathan intended to follow the technique he and Gareth had developed on their 'hover-hearse' trip from Emeti. Michael later confessed he would have been much more concerned about their situation had it not been for his knowledge of the success of that trip.

A VHF radio had recently been fitted to the *Dr Andrew*. While it transmitted satisfactorily over a long distance, perversely it would not receive properly except within a few hundred yards (metres) of the transmitter. Heading downriver, Jonathan radioed Awaba to relay a message to Balimo that they were on their way. Having no way of knowing if the message was being received, he repeated it at intervals. Calling in at Awaba they learned from Russell Peake that Balimo had the message and had replied, asking that they stop overnight at Kawito. They would be joined there the next day by the *Jean Goodman* and the rest of the team for the Ali venture. After a day of handling oily drums of diesel, changing finger ties in the mud, hauling out grass from under the skirt and generally heaving about the hovercraft in the heat, the offer of a shower at the Tuckers' sounded like bliss.

With the best of intentions, Brian Black contacted them there by radio. He knew that they had intended to return to Balimo before setting off on the Ali trip and thought there might be some kit that Jonathan and Martin would need to bring out the next day. Michael, too, would now be stranded at Kawito until the return of the two craft from Ali, and he also might need some belongings.

Jonathan and Martin soon listed their needs, but with Michael it was rather different. Unused to the radio routine and not being a man of few words he went into considerable detail about his needs, even to a full description of the colour and pattern of the pyjamas he required. The transmission was an open one and could be heard all the way from Saiwasi to Awaba; nor could Brian cut in, for it was single-direction speech only. According to Brian the whole procedure took twenty-five minutes. For a good deal of that time Michael was chattering away to himself unheard by anyone, as the radio automatically cut off transmission after a short period. The process totally clogged up the Balimo radio and blocked any other transmissions. 'Over' and 'out' were clearly not in Michael's vocabulary.

The position was reversed when Brian came to assemble the requested items. Michael's were easily located, thanks to his tidiness; with Jonathan and Martin it was quite a different matter. With a sleeping Ben contributing to the clutter in the room the three of them shared, it was a major task of discovery, taking until long after midnight before Brian completed his collection. Falling into bed he set his alarm for 4.15 am. Breakfast was to be at 5 am for a six o'clock start for Ali.

Maybe they were not fully awake at that early hour but the Balimo group had hardly been on the way more than ten minutes before *Jean Goodman* was aground in the lagoon. With Gareth jumping up and down on the nose of the craft and Brian sloshing about in the water, Gordon managed to drive off, and they continued without further incident. Chris Hooke the cameraman and Lindsay Dodd the sound recordist followed in the aluminium dinghy so they could capture events from the trip. After topping up to the brim with fuel at Kawito the convoy set out; Gordon and

Brian in *Jean Goodman*, Gareth, Jenny and Jonathan in *Dr Andrew* and Martin Healey and the film crew in the dinghy. The two hovercraft had benefited from the engineers' attentions and were performing well; they had to throttle back to allow the film boat to keep up.

Approaching Awaba, they passed the cattle barge going downriver. Simply crossing the wake of the barge was enough to pull out three finger ties on the rear corner of the *Dr Andrew*. The ease with which the ties continued to break was becoming a matter for concern. For the moment there was nothing more they could do about it except to pause briefly at Awaba to replace the ties. Soon they reached the lagoon short cut. With Jonathan leading, they set off to navigate the lagoon. The dinghy could not cope with the weed as the propeller of the outboard repeatedly clogged, even though Jonathan attempted to follow the maze of interconnecting channels rather than keeping to the straight hovercraft route. Transferring the film crew to *Jean Goodman* Martin left in the dinghy to follow the river route to Makapa.

The diversion from the previous day's route was part of their undoing; had they kept to it everything might have gone well. Confident in the precision of the GPS Jonathan set off to find the exit from the lagoon. To his dismay he found that in their exhilaration the previous day the intrepid navigators had failed to record the actual position of the exit they had hit with such unfailing accuracy. For the next hour, the two hovercraft chased up and down long stretches of the lagoon, searching for the narrow, fast-flowing channel to the exit, their every blundering effort being recorded by the amused film crew. Time and again they stopped to compare GPS readings, consult maps, and take bearings on the position shown on the map for the lagoon exit.

Admitting defeat, they backtracked to the lagoon entrance and set off the long way round, following the river as Martin had done.

The exit from the lagoon still existed; they had almost begun to doubt it. From the river the exit was clear to see. Checking its position by GPS they found it was 766 yards (700 metres) from the location shown on the map; all their bearings had been aiming at the wrong point. Assuming the maps were correct in the first place, over the years change had taken place in the river system. It was important to check and record data as each new route was found. Memory and line of sight cannot be relied on in this terrain; channels are almost invisible from the lagoon until one is virtually right on top of them.

Martin had travelled along the river towards the exit from the lagoon, expecting to see the two hovercraft waiting for him, but there was no sign of them. He decided to go a little further upriver before stopping to wait at a landing point close to a small shelter hut. As Martin approached he noticed a woman working in a riverside garden nearby. By the time he had tied up the boat she had disappeared.

Following the river after Martin the hovercraft stopped at Makapa to refuel from the barrel dropped off the previous day. The crews were told that Martin had gone further along the river. One of the pastors at Makapa offered to show them another exit from the lagoon on the northern side, which would put them further on the way to Ali, so cutting out another section of the river. He was used to thinking in terms of canoe widths, as they found. The channel narrowed more and more the further they went, so at one point it was little more than a quarter the width of the craft. It twisted and turned in a way that more than tested the drivers' skill.

Within sight of the river, the inevitable happened again: both hovercraft became stuck in a patch of tall dense vegetation more like sugar cane than the reeds they had been used to. Half an hour later with help from the villagers and the usual soaking for the crew, they rejoined Martin upstream on the river where they had a much-needed lunch. Shortly after the arrival of the hovercraft a man appeared with a small boy. He was yet another of the local pastors and the brother of the bashful woman who had vanished when Martin had landed. The pastor explained that as a lone woman it was not acceptable for her to meet a man on his own, but had there been two or more men it would have been fine. It was a reminder that care had to be taken not to overstep the local mores.

Shortly after passing the junction between the Soari and the Aramia rivers, Gordon decided they should stop and set up camp for the night. In an area cleared by their grass knives, the crews lit a campfire with wood collected from the surrounding forest. Beans, chicken curry and instant potato from the 1989 compo packs were washed down with a welcome cup of tea. The food tasted surprisingly palatable, despite its great age. It was not long before the local equivalent of a pizza delivery service arrived. A passing group of Gogodala men pulled in their canoe and, after greetings, offered to barter some large freshwater prawns they had just caught in the river in return for 'smokes'. They had picked the wrong commodity, but Gordon soon traded some packets of rice and sugar from the compo rations instead. Thrown on the fire the prawns quickly turned from grey to bright pink and proved to be deliciously succulent, rounding off the meal well. Shortly another helping arrived. A second canoe pulled in, sent by Stuart Henderson's son. Stuart, a New Zealander, had settled many years before near Makapa and he and his son were obviously well tuned in to the local bush telegraph. More prawns were traded and quickly followed the first batch before everyone settled down for the night.

Nets draped over the open 'gull-wing' cabin doors and seats folded flat quickly converted the hovercraft into reasonably mosquito-free sleeping areas for their crews. Martin preferred to bed down in the dinghy with a net over him, and the film crew used the tents they had brought. After a wash in the river, and shortly before the light had gone completely, they were all bedded down. It was just 6.30 pm. Sleep did not come easily for some at that early hour. The forest was far from quiet: droning mosquitoes, chirruping cicadas and some unfamiliar noises were disturbing. The strange surroundings and the consciousness of the unknown just 'out there' did not help, nor did local noise by way of snores. Every sound seemed magnified in the still night air and distant noises were reflected over the water. In the darkness, each sudden noise seemed a potential threat, whether from land or water.

Brian had taken a long time to get off to sleep. When he woke the darkness was lightened by the moon. He knew sleep would not return but he lay as still as possible for a long time, not wishing to disturb the others. Eventually his patience ran out and he had to get up. He crept, or so he thought, under the net and along the deck onto the river bank. Later Gareth pointedly told him it was only 4.10 am; moored side by side, the two hovercraft were touching, and the movement of one disturbed Gareth in the other.

The ashes of the fire soon revived, which was cheery, but quickly Brian realised his great mistake in leaving the comparative safety of the netted hovercraft. Everyone else might be asleep, but the mosquitoes most certainly were not: they were rampant. In his efforts to assemble kit for others the previous night he had failed to pack long-sleeved shirt and long trousers for himself. Clad only in short-sleeved shirt and shorts he was a wonderful target for the voracious mossies, which made the most of the opportunity. On getting back to base he counted fifty-three bites on the front and side of one leg alone. His state of mind was not helped when Gordon appeared at 5 am and said, 'When you got up you let in a squadron of mossies.'

A couple of miles upriver from the campsite the river made a large, sweeping loop. At the narrow neck of the loop little more than five yards (metres) separated the two channels as the water-course turned back on itself. Here the locals had made a significant short cut by digging a channel through the narrow bank between the two lengths of the river. The water pouring through the narrow man-made channel built up into a very minor rapid, because of the constriction rather than due to any difference in level. Compared to the very real and hazardous rapids encountered on the China expedition, this flow did not even warrant the name. So flat is the whole of the Fly area that the gradient of the river is no more than 1 in 800,000. For the fun of it the craft were taken through the strong flow a few times. Even though Ali was now only about nineteen miles (thirty kilometres) upriver, Gordon calculated that they did not have enough fuel in reserve to reach Ali and get back to Kawito, where the rest of the fuel was stored. They had been defeated because it had been impossible to get enough diesel to Makapa. For future medical patrols to Ali, it would be necessary to extend the range of the craft by having larger supplies at Makapa so the craft could be refuelled on both outward and return journeys. Another operational requirement for the future had been established.

On the return journey, *Jean Goodman* with Gordon driving,

was in the lead and going well. Jonathan, following in *Dr Andrew*, noticed that the lead craft had slowed down up ahead. He assumed it was to enable him to catch up, and he opened up to full speed. Approaching at full throttle Jonathan realised too late what had happened. On a deceptively tight right-hand bend Gordon had swung wide and gone into the reeds on the outside bank. There the craft was stuck and the *Jean* was bearing down on the same path, in danger of crashing into the stranded craft.

Already turning into the bend, Jonathan slammed on full right elevon. He wrestled with the rudder to stop the rear end sliding out like a car skidding on ice. Gareth grabbed Jenny and hurled their collective weight to the far right side of the cabin. The craft banked at an impossibly steep angle as the right-hand side of the skirt clawed at the water to get a grip and they shot past the other craft with no more than a yard (metre) to spare. As they did so Jonathan saw Gordon grinning widely as he gave a big thumbs-up sign in relief.

Both craft lost a few rear finger ties as a result of the incident so they beached on a small mudbank to do repairs. Scrambling around on the slippery deck Brian lost his footing and for the umpteenth time in two days found himself soaked from head to foot. While the repairs were under way Martin took the dinghy ahead so the film crew could get some coverage of the riverside wildlife. Shortly, the rest were to see a little more of that than they wished.

Repairs completed they set off, this time with Gareth driving *Jean Goodman* so he could compare the performance of the two craft. Even with the benefit of the previous day's experience they did not find the short cut through the lagoon the first time. On one of the false trails, Jonathan managed to get his craft stranded on a floating mass of dead grass. The only way to deal with this hazard was for the crew to jump over the side and tread on the grass until it sank below the surface to enable the skirt to seal on the water. Martin was doing that at the front while Jonathan juggled with the controls to try to rock the craft free. Glancing down to the right through the open door Jonathan saw a poisonous snake, a taipan, slither out from under the craft directly beneath him and head up through the grass towards the front of the craft. Martin was now walking back along the deck towards the open door. 'Snake!' Jonathan shouted, and pointed at the grass. Wearing earplugs against the noise, Martin misunderstood the gesture. He thought more grass treading was needed and obligingly jumped over the side. He landed where Jonathan was pointing — exactly where the snake had been seen only a second before. Gordon and Jonathan screamed at full pitch 'Snake!' That got through! With an expression of total horror Martin jumped from the grass mat in one great leap onto the deck of the craft landing in a crumpled but otherwise unharmed heap. It had been too close for comfort.

On the way downriver Gareth, driving with every cell of his body as only he can, had coaxed 30.9 knots out of one of the craft, a record on water for the expedition; Graeme had achieved 31 knots over mudbanks. Allowing for the climatic conditions this was well up to the specified performance and showed that the engineers had done much to overcome the early problems. But if somehow even more thrust could be found, it would help cope with the more taxing conditions of travelling upriver against the current and in the face of a stiff wind. For six months of the year the south-easterly trade winds can blow at speeds of up to twenty or even twenty-five knots.

It was difficult to see how more power could be produced.

Already the engineers had made adjustments to the angle of the blades of the thrust fans. That had certainly produced an improvement but there was nothing more that could be gained in that way. The engines had been 'tweaked' and adjusted to top performance, yet still the engineers were not entirely satisfied. Maybe engineers are always like that. Steve, in particular, had the nagging thought that they had not taken some factor into account despite all that had been achieved.

Gordon's estimate of the fuel range had been right. As they approached Kawito both craft were on the last of the fuel in their second tanks. The first had long since been emptied. Settling on the river bank at Kawito they waited for the required two minutes to allow the turbocharger to cool before switching off the engines. As they did so, the fuel gauge in Jonathan's craft clicked against the zero stop. They had just made it. With the craft refuelled and the crews refreshed by a snack provided by the Tuckers, they headed for Balimo, the Ali adventure over.

There was less than a week to go now for the eleven remaining members of the total team of twenty-five. Most of the tasks left were in preparation for departure so there would inevitably be an air of 'running down' from now on. But before they could feel any sense of anticlimax they had a tremendous boost from the medical missionary staff. On the final Sunday evening there was a joint farewell party at the nurses' home for the team and Jill Adams, who would shortly be returning home. The team were wearing white tee shirts specially screen-printed in Balimo; they had been given by Celestine in appreciation of the hovercraft and the team's work. Printed on the front of the shirts was the team logo and the words 'Wings of Love and Life'. It was a festive occasion and the nurses put on some entertainment with much singing, drama and lots of fun. The food was supplied jointly by the nurses, the medical staff and the team, but the latter were able to relax as guests and enjoy themselves without having to do the work. Many thanks were expressed to the expedition for their efforts and their friendship. Gordon was able to reply, expressing our appreciation of the great welcome we had been given and the friendship shown to us. Rightly he said that Balimo and everyone associated with it would be fondly remembered by the team for a long time to come. It was a very happy final gathering.

Steve Moody was still not satisfied with the hovercraft. Although both craft were now performing well, something was still niggling away at his mind. Ilaba, Dekame, Sebia and Olo, the four national hovercraft drivers, arrived as Steve was writing a report for HoverAid. They had a similar feeling and wanted to review with him some of the problems in operating the craft. Time was running out, as Steve would be leaving in a few days. They ran over some of the problems: the earlier overheating of the engine, the strain on the thrust fan belts and pulleys and the ease with which finger ties were repeatedly torn out, always on the rear corners of the skirt.

As they went through these and other items, a pattern started to form in Steve's mind. He realised with a flash of insight that there could be a common cause. The engineers had adjusted the angle of the thrust fan blades to get more power to push the hovercraft forward, but they had not really thought about what might be holding it back. He remembered the abandoned trip to Pikewa Creek. Performance had been low and afterwards the engineers found a sheet of foam underneath the craft had been causing some drag. What if that had simply been extra drag? Could the craft have been suffering drag all the way through? They certainly hadn't been like that on trials in the UK, but was there a factor in PNG they had overlooked?

The four drivers and Steve talked it over excitedly. On the Fly trip he had thought the craft were lower in the water than he expected. Could the less dense hot air of the tropics be reducing the skirt pressure and so not giving enough lift? If so, that would create drag and account for many of the problems. It seemed too simple to be the answer and they decided to experiment. It was not difficult to alter the angle of the lift fan blades to suck more air into the skirt but the effect delighted the engineers. The craft sat up on an increased cushion of air and at once it was much lighter on the controls and more powerful. The difference was remarkable. It was so dramatic that they were able to reduce the earlier adjustment to the thrust fans and get a better balance of power between lift and forward push.

It was a gratifying result. Only a couple of days before the end of the project, they had produced the effect Steve was seeking. They had already got the craft performing well, but now they were even better; well up to specification, possibly over it, given the tropical conditions. With a full passenger and equipment load there was still good performance, and the craft were very easy to manoeuvre. Steve felt they could now leave with confidence, knowing that the craft were well up to the job they had been brought out to do.

At the hover-garage there were still a few things to do: final coats of oil to be applied to the boarding, tools to be stacked or returned if borrowed. Brian completed his bargemaster duties by finding willing buyers for some surplus items of equipment. A quantity of clothing that many of the team members had decided to leave behind was very gratefully received at Mapodo. The last of the roofing iron was placed on the church, finishing off a job outstanding from its original construction almost two years before. Surplus food found its way into many local larders. Finally items of furniture supplied from the missionary homes to make our stay more comfortable were returned and items shuffled between Patterson's and Lagoon View were redistributed as we found them.

Wednesday 12 May saw the departure of the film crew. The two Chrises, Lindsay and Mike had been living with the team for a month and had shared in the chores as well as the adventures. They had put up with our quirky ways and we had tried to meet their professional needs with as easy a grace as was possible. We looked forward to seeing the result of their work and hoped that we had not made complete fools of ourselves too often in front of the cameras.

Gordon, too, left later the same day to start the wind down from the Port Moresby end and to arrange the details of the team's return flights. Due to the involvement of RAAF planes in Somalia, the team could not take advantage of free passage on a Hercules training flight. That meant additional cost on our already strained budget and Gordon hoped to find ways of keeping that to a minimum. There were many other financial and administrative matters that Bruce Olsen had been handling for us that Gordon had to settle before the team left Moresby.

There remained only the final departure but first Brian was seen off in a special way. He decided he would take a photograph of the cassowary bird which wandered around the place. After some stalking he located it on the lagoon shore near the council chamber. Camera at the ready, he approached the apparently indifferent bird and took a snapshot. Encouraged by his success he moved closer. This, the cassowary decided, was being over-familiar and it started towards Brian aggressively. Clearly it had a different kind of closeup in mind; so Brian decided to retreat. As the bird quickened its approach so he too speeded up, heading for a small clump of trees that might provide cover. Faced by a steep bank on which the bird might well outperform him Brian threw dignity away and made a run for it, urged on by some delighted spectators. After a 200-yard (about 200-metre) sprint he looked back, only to find that the bird had lost interest in its fleeing quarry and he was safe from yet another of the perils of Papua.

The farewells started early on the final day. While the team were still doing final packing and making a last attempt to tidy up Patterson's there was a steady stream of callers. Many of the nurses, hospital staff and missionaries dropped in to say goodbye. Finally everything was assembled outside Patterson's for one last tractor ride to the airstrip. While it was good to be heading home after more than two and a half months away, leaving was not easy. So much had been shared, so many new relationships had been made, so much had happened that leaving Balimo was a wrench. We had done all we intended to do, and the hovercraft were in place. But like a parent leaving a child it was not easy to walk away. Thoughts of how the hovercraft service was running, of the difficulties the drivers would be facing, of the way in which it would be affecting the lives of people in the riverside villages would remain with us. There was a sense in which something of each of us would still be at Balimo.

'Hovercraft Expedition says Goodbye and Thank You to Balimo' read the poster on the back of the tractor trailer as the team pulled out. Many of the Gogodala were travelling out on the trailer in addition to the team so they could say a final farewell at the airstrip. The following pick-up truck driven by Graham Tucker was also packed with people. More were making their way on foot along the road out to the airstrip. So waves and greetings were constantly being exchanged. There was plenty of time for everyone to gather, for the Ok Tedi Mining Company plane was late arriving. The last goodbyes were said, hugs exchanged, tears wiped from eyes and cheeks as the plane door closed. As the plane taxied out and then sped down the runway, hands and handkerchiefs fluttered in final waves. Then the team were airborne and on their way.

The crew of the small plane made their way to their seats with difficulty. Every possible nook and cranny was crammed with backpacks, bags and packages. A fair amount of the Kini carvers' work over the last month or so had found its way on to the plane, too, as souvenirs of our stay. The pilot had been staggered at the amount of kit to be packed; no doubt mining company executives travel lighter than hovercraft project teams. We were grateful to Ok Tedi. Thanks to the help of the company the team and the baggage were being flown out free of charge.

It was a clear day with light broken cloud. As the plane gained height Balimo Health Centre and the settlement could be seen spread out below. The lagoon system and many places beyond the lagoon where we had ventured were in view too. The extravagant loops of the Aramia stood out clearly, sweeping across the flat floodplain below as far behind as the eye could see and on to the Bamu, as our flight progressed further west. The great width of the Bamu was dwarfed as it flowed into the mighty Fly, which in turn lost itself in the expanse of the Gulf of Papua.

Soon Port Moresby loomed ahead and the team made its last touchdown in PNG. This was the last time, too, that the remainder of the team would be together for from here they were going off in different directions — Cairns, Brisbane and Sydney.

Once more the team packed into the mission houses and enjoyed the hospitality of the Olsen family. The Olsens took the team to see the crocodiles being fed at the wildlife park. We had managed to avoid feeding them in the Fly area, and here everyone could safely feel very brave about it. A highlight of the Moresby stay was the informal supper given by the British High Commissioner, John Guy. He had taken a great interest in the expedition and had helped in many ways. Later he was to write, 'I thought the project a tremendous success. The team members brought great credit to Britain and I was immensely gratified to have been associated with the venture.'

On the final evening the team gave a thank you supper to the Olsens and all the missionary folk of the ECP who had been involved with the project. It was quite a gathering, very fittingly rounded off as once again we enjoyed Ron Smith's talent on the electronic organ as we had done on our very first evening in Port Moresby. Although we had not planned it that way we had arrived in PNG on a Sunday. Now the team was leaving on the Lord's Day, too; that seemed very appropriate.

Epilogue

Maidame died, Kubili lived. That is a matter of record, which encapsulates the work of the expedition. Our aim was to help an operation in place long before we appeared on the scene, and on which much depends for the future. We set out to provide a new service that would enable the work of the Balimo Health Centre to be even more effective in the future. We wanted also to encourage others by showing what hovercraft can do so that they might have the hope and ambition to stretch out to help people elsewhere in new ways.

So, does our project have significance for the future or is it now simply history?

A group of individuals, mostly strangers to each other, were brought together through the efforts of one man, Mike Cole. Together they worked to raise funds for the project and received the help of many people and some organisations. Two hovercraft were bought, transported across the globe and assembled in Papua New Guinea. They have been tested and tried and shown to be well up to the demanding task of aiding a much-needed hospital working on limited resources. A trained and competent national team of operators now have the craft and are gaining in operational experience. Their work needs nurturing and supporting while it takes root and matures. That, too, is part of the continuing work of the project.

At the time of writing Gordon Goodman, the leader of the expedition in the field, is preparing to return to Papua New Guinea in September for a brief visit. He will take out parts and modifications for the hovercraft and review progress with the hospital team. He will be giving them support and encouragement as well as bringing back first-hand operational news to supporters and to the expedition team, which meets again in October. Meanwhile at the hospital a volunteer is working alongside the medical superintendent to relieve him of many of the practical day-to-day tasks involved in running the hospital. That work includes supporting and providing oversight to the four nationals who are now responsible for the operation of the hovercraft service.

HoverAid is actively assimilating the reports of the expedition engineers and applying the operational experience gained to its continuing work of helping people in developing countries overcome problems of communications and transportation. The HoverAid designers and engineers are also continuing to work on possible further improvements to the PNG machines. Early in 1994 two engineers will visit Balimo as part of that process, conferring with the national team.

Andrew Schache, one of the two Queenslanders who were members of the expedition, has applied to the Evangelical Church of Papua New Guinea to join the mission team at Balimo as the hospital maintenance engineer. He is currently raising financial support to enable him to do that and expects to be at Balimo early in 1994. The hospital has been without a maintenance engineer for two years and the load has been carried by the medical superintendent. Amongst Andrew's duties will be overseeing the hovercraft service, bringing to that work the range of experience he gained as a member of the expedition and the benefit of his continuing links with his fellow members and their supporters.

It wasn't all hard slog on the expedition. We had great fun, too.

We laughed and cried together; relaxed and marvelled together; enjoyed worship together; made new and lasting friendships. Our antics provided considerable entertainment for the Gogodala as we sometimes floundered around. We gained the sense of achievement that comes from completing challenging tasks and learning new skills. None of us came back unchanged; the memories of the shared fun and joy alone ensure that.

Mike Cole continues to take forward the concept of using the small River Rover hovercraft for medical work in places where the conditions and the means do not allow any other form of help. Currently he is in Nicaragua carrying out a reconnaissance for a possible future expedition.

The hover-ambulance service is now available at Balimo and beyond the lagoon. It will continue to need support as part of the work of the ECP in running the Balimo Health Centre.

We have played our small part. We went in Christ's Name and to Him we commit what has been done.

Appendix A
Hoverdoctor Expedition: Diary of Events

8 May 1989
Balimo and Mapodo, Papua New Guinea
Australian mission doctor Graham Zerk shares concern for reaching remote Gogodala people with medical services with UK colleague, Helen Brackenbury.

Dr Zerk reads *Journey to the Fourth World* is inspired by Dr Bill Gould's hoverdoctor vision and writes to Squadron Leader Michael Cole.

October 1989
Gorsley, UK
Helen Brackenbury on UK leave confirms the hoverdoctor need to Michael Cole.

5 - 9 December 1989
Hong Kong, then Papua New Guinea
Michael Cole diverts from his final China expedition recce to visit Graham Zerk and the Fly River area. MAF provides aerial recce of area.

July - August 1990
Balimo and Fly River area
Captain Tony Sewell, member of the China expedition team is sent to Fly River area and spends one month thoroughly exploring the possibilities. Plans for hoverdoctor service with Dr Andrew Baur and Dr Graham Zerk are put in place. Mission engineer Laurie Humphrey plans the hover-garage.

22 October - 9 November 1991
Gorsley and Salisbury to PNG
Dr Rachel Pinniger and Jeff Goulding visit PNG, seeking to renew the vision.

Sunday 3 March 1992
Balimo and Mapodo, PNG
Michael Cole travels to Latin America via Papua New Guinea. At Balimo Mission Hospital on Sunday 3 March it takes all day for boy with snakebite to reach Balimo Hospital from remote village. He dies. In consultation with Dr Graham Tucker the resolve to go forward is firmly made.

25 July 1992
Linton, Herefordshire, UK
The expedition team, mixture of youth and maturity, assembles for the first time. Two HoverAid River Rover hovercraft are to be purchased. Michael Cole hands field leadership to Wing Commander Gordon Goodman.

2 September 1992
Tari, PNG
Formal permission is granted for expedition to go ahead.

24 February 1993
Heathrow, UK
The main expedition team leaves for Papua New Guinea.

13 March 1993
Kawito, PNG
The first hovercraft *Dr Andrew Baur* is launched in PNG. Crew: Michael Cole, Dick Bell, Dr Bill Gould, Gordon Goodman.

8 April 1993
Port Moresby harbour, PNG
The second River Rover hovercraft *Jean Goodman* arrives and gives a public display in the harbour of Port Moresby.

29 - 30 April 1993
Fly River delta, PNG
Both River Rover hovercraft explore remote mudflat areas of the Fly River delta with Dr Graham Zerk on board.

5 May 1993
Balimo Hospital, PNG
Formal handover of hovercraft and hover-garage to Dr Graham Tucker, superintendent of Balimo Hospital. Witnessed by H. E. Francis Koimanrea, Minister for Health; Mr Kuok Bitan, MP; John Guy, OBE, British High Commissioner; and expedition team.

15 July 1993
Brisbane, Australia
Australian team member Andrew Schache confirms his willingness to return to Balimo to be the permanent hover-doctor service manager.

Appendix B
PNG Hovercraft Team
February to May 1993

UK Members

Squadron Leader
Bob Abbott, MBE
(UK liaison)
Jonathan Allan
Squadron Leader
Dick Bell
Brian Black
Aileen Boyd
Squadron Leader
Michael Cole, OBE
Martin Fairley
Barbara Fergusson
John Field
Wing Commander
Gordon Goodman
Dr Bill Gould
Jeff Goulding (recce)
Timothy Goulding
Martin Healey
Amanda Lee
Steve Moody
Squadron Leader
Donald Moreland
(UK treasurer)
Ben Oliver
Cecil Pearse
Michael Pinkess
Dr Rachel Pinniger
Captain Tony Shewell (recce)
Gareth Smith
Sarah Williams

Australia and New Zealand Members
Flying Officer
Graeme Bencke, RAF
Flight Lieutenant
Rachel Grimmer, RAAF
Laurie Humphrey
Bruce Olsen
Andrew Schache
Jenny Smith
Ron Smith
Dr Graham Tucker
Dr Graham Zerk

John Gau TV Production Crew
Chris Powell, Producer
Chris Hooke,
Director/Cameraman
Lindsay Dodd, Sound
Recordist
Michael Robinson, Assistant
Cameraman

U.K. TEAM MEMBERS - February to May 1993

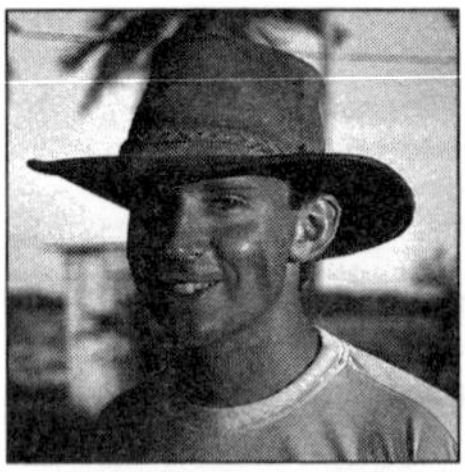
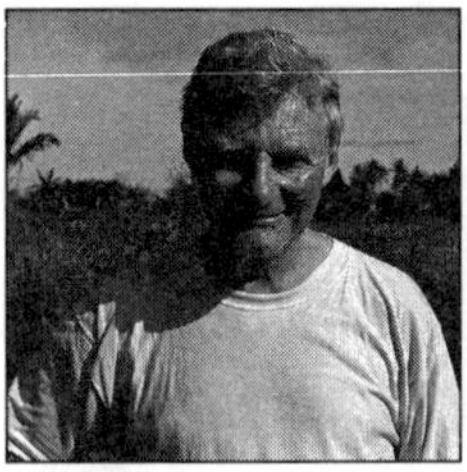
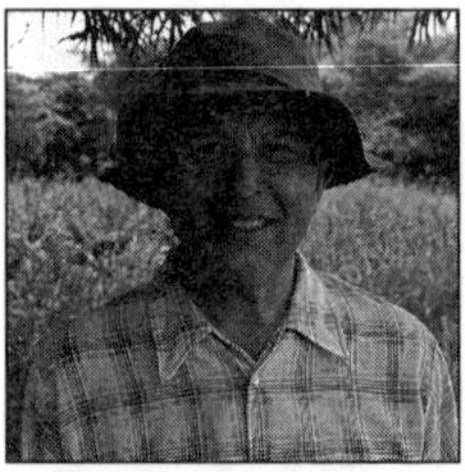

Left to right: Jonathan Allan, Squadron Leader Dick Bell, Brian Black

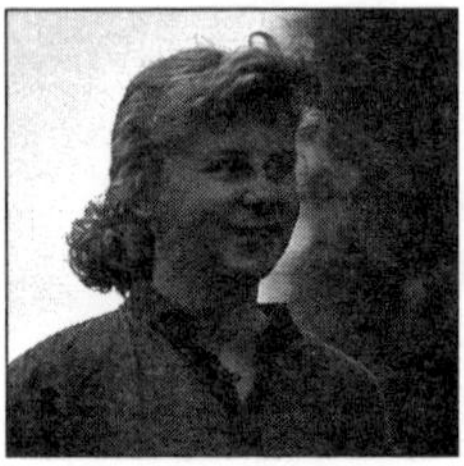
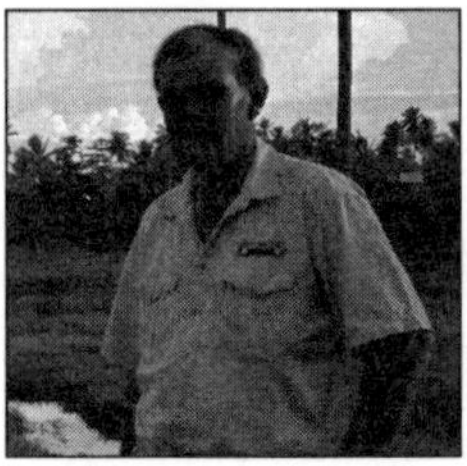
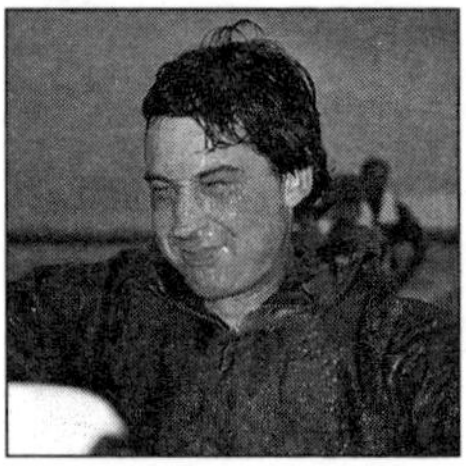

Left to right: Aileen Boyd, Squadron Leader Michael Cole OBE, Martin Fairley

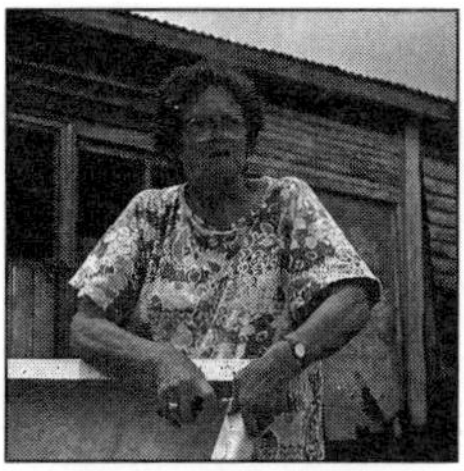
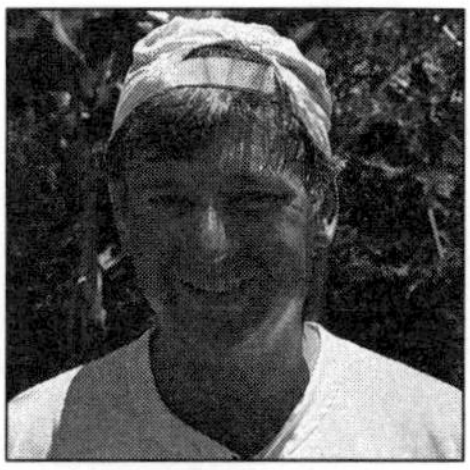
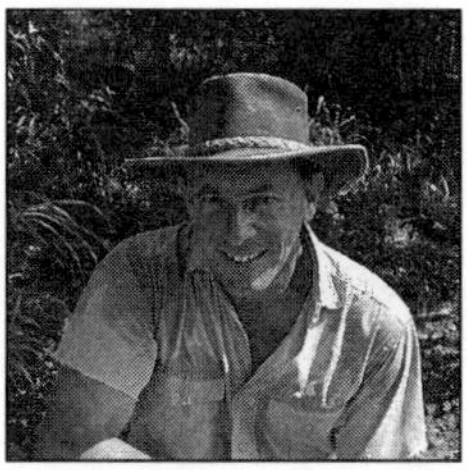

Left to right: Barbara Fergusson, John Field, Wing Commander Gordon Goodman

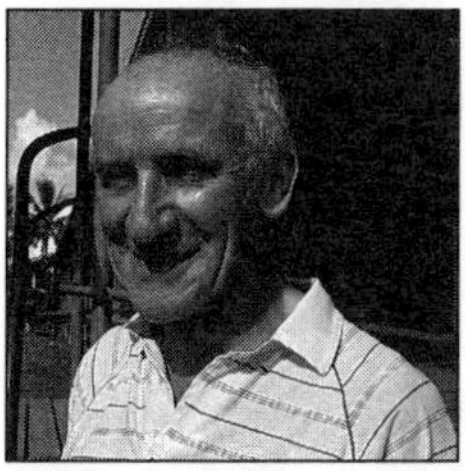
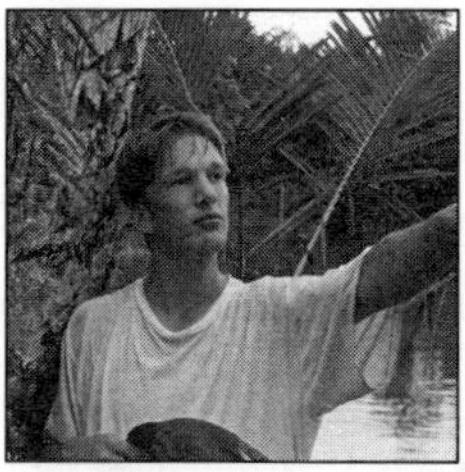
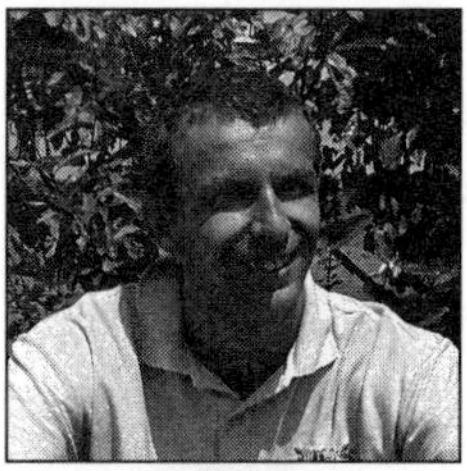

Left to right: Dr Bill Gould, Timothy Goulding, Martin Healey

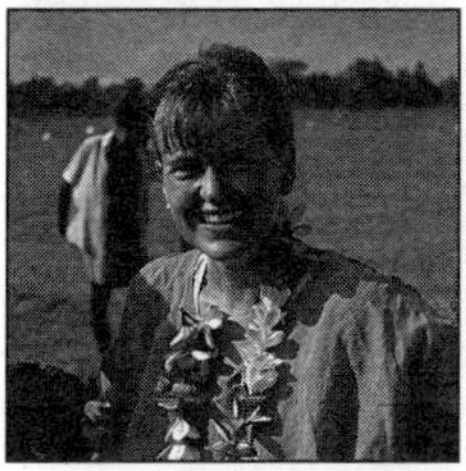
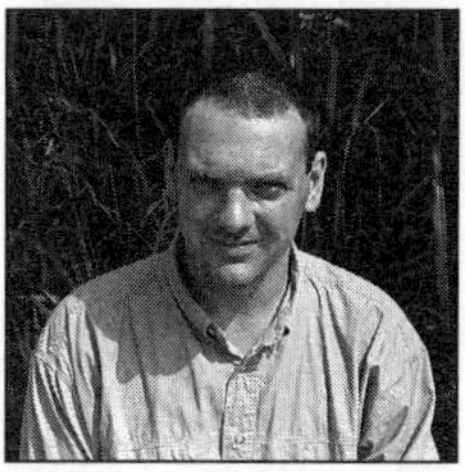
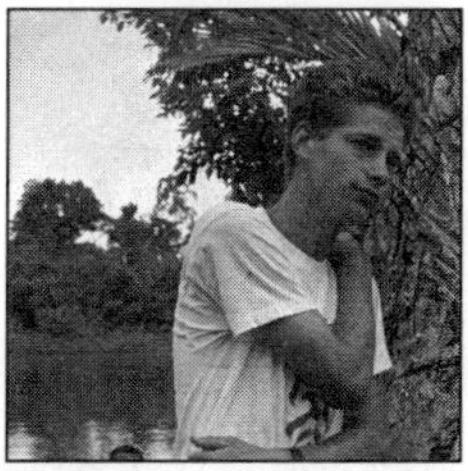

Left to right: Amanda Lee, Steve Moody, Ben Oliver

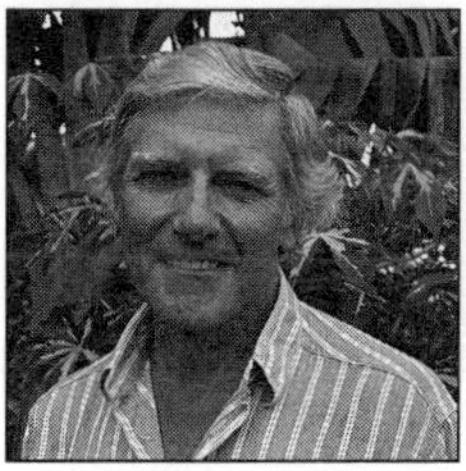
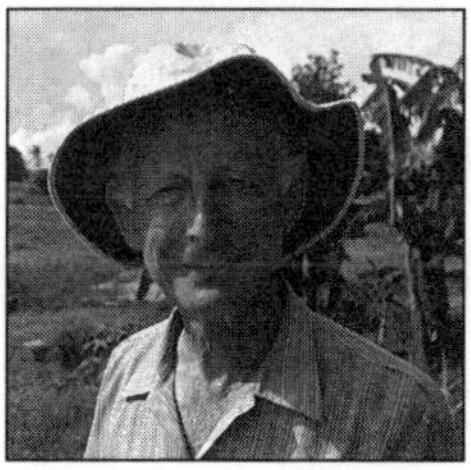
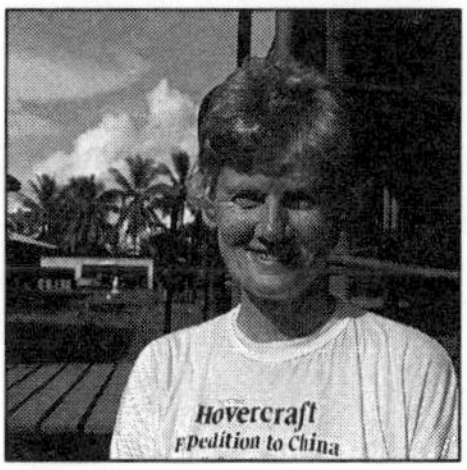

Left to right: Cecil Pearse(author), Michael Pinkness, Dr Rachel Pinniger

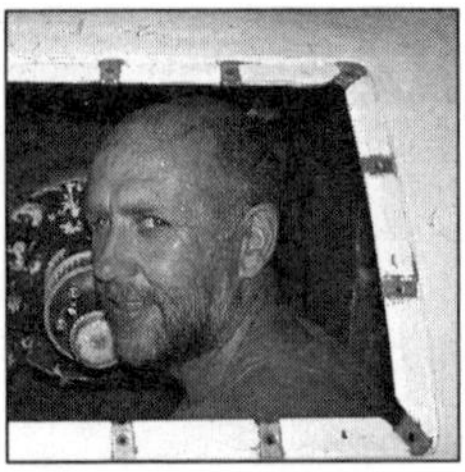
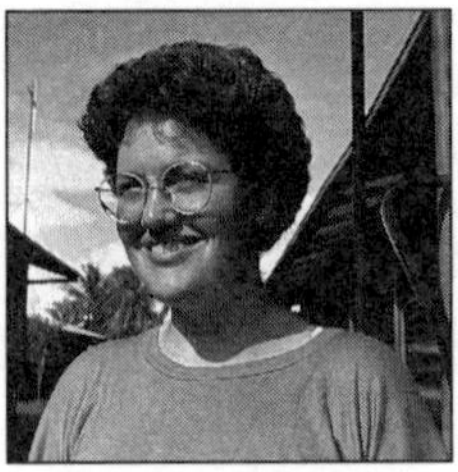

Left to right: Gareth Smith, Sarah Williams

AUSTRALIAN /NEW ZEALAND TEAM MEMBERS - February to May 1993

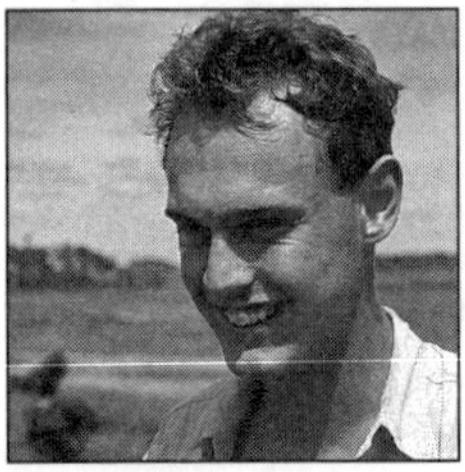
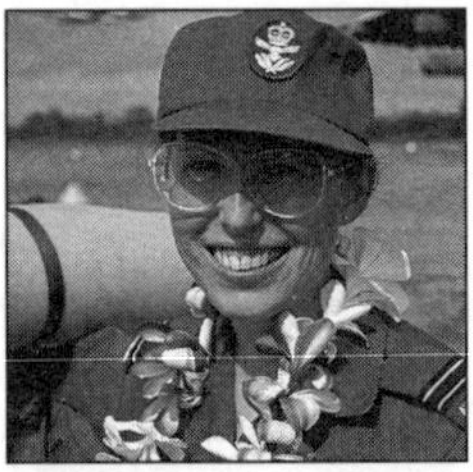
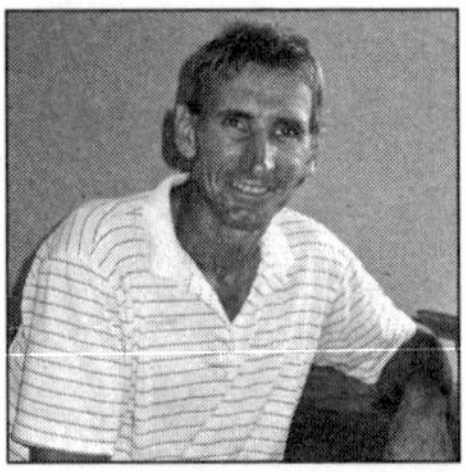

Left to right: Flying Officer Graeme Bencke RAF, Flight Lieutenant (Dr) Rachel Grimmer RAAF, Laurie Humphrey

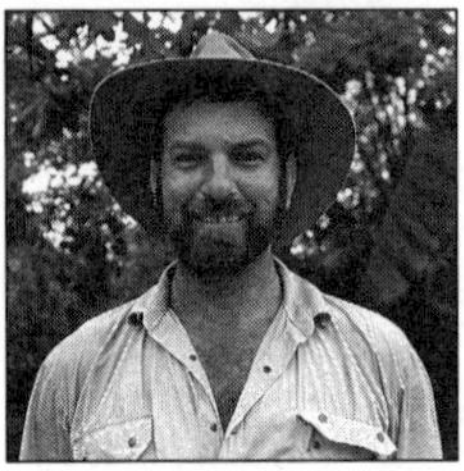
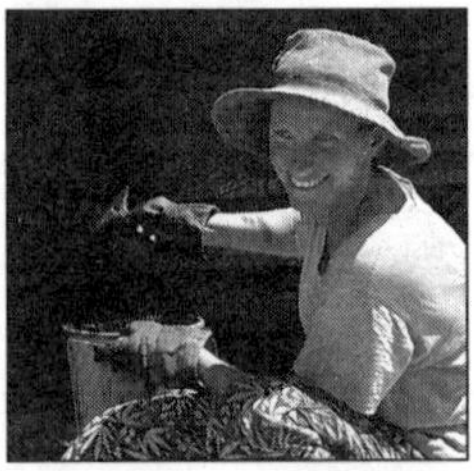
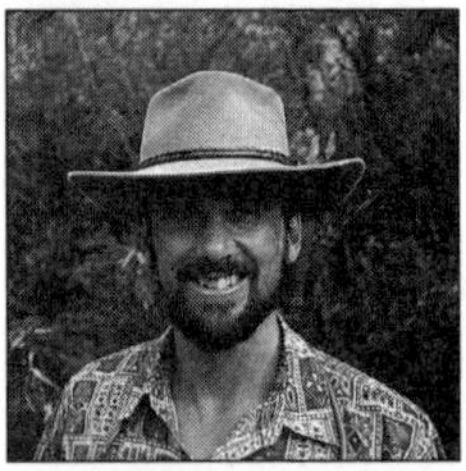

Left to right: Andrew Schache, Jenny Smith, Dr Graham Zerk

Appendix C
Supporters

Major Supporters
Mr Philip J. Baur, Jr, Philadephia, USA
Mr Kenneth Hugh Goodman, Wellington, Somerset, UK

Supporters
Mr Peter Atkins
Mr & Mrs Bob Arnold
Mrs N. Avery
Mrs Rachel Baird
Mr & Mrs P. Bailey
Mrs M. Bevan
Mr & Mrs Ian Barlow
Mrs Elizabeth Bird
Wg-Cdr and Mrs S. D. Baldock
Miss Irene Bailey
Dr & Mrs R. F. J. Cole
Mr M Cadbury
Mr A. D. Currie
Mr. K. Currie
Mr & Mrs J. H. Cole
Sqn-Ldr & Mrs D. Childs
Mr & Mrs Crofton
Mr & Mrs Arthur Cheetham
Mrs Brenda Cook
Mr John Craggs
Mr & Mrs Bethany-Cox
Miss Cynthia Craddock
Mr & Mrs Roy Craddock
Mr M. A. Cracknell
Mr. M. Dunne
Mrs. T. B. Davis
Mr Dickson
Mr & Mrs Richard Dew
Mr & Mrs Alistair Dowell
Mr & Mrs Richard Evans
Mrs W. A. Field
Miss Helen Fleet
Mr J. Garrett
Mr & Mrs A. Golding
Mr John Guy, OBE
Mr & Mrs Peter Grealis
Lt Col G. Groom
Mrs Sarah Goulding
Mrs Annabel Goodhal
Mrs Marion Green

Mrs E. Hall
Mr C. Harley
Miss M. Harris
Mrs M. Hazell
Miss T. Hunt
Rt Hon Sir Edward Heath, KG, MBE, MP
The Viscountess Head
Sqn-Ldr M. T. Holdsworth
Mr & Mrs Heath
Mr & Mrs Peter Hoffman
Mrs J. Henderson
Mr Andy Harris
Mr Brian Harrison
Mr & Mrs Hoskisson
Mr Peter Johnson
Mr & Mrs Rupert Judge
Miss Lilian James
Mr & Mrs Francis King
Mr & Mrs Deil Kopharmel
Mr & Mrs Arthur Kelsall
Mr J. Lancaster
Sir Desmond and Lady Lee
Mr & Mrs Martin Lee
Mr & Mrs Gordon Lillie
Mr & Mrs Derek Leek
Mr & Mrs Steve Leek
Mr & Mrs Bernard Lewis
Mr & Mrs Tim Longley
Miss Fiona Leyland
Mr D. Martin
Sir Carol Mather
Mr R. Mills
Mr P. Mitchell
Mr Barry Myers
Mr & Mrs John Millard
Mr & Mrs Mark Mitchell
Rev A. Mackay
Mr Patrick McGeorge
Mr & Mrs George Mounter
Mr & Mrs Gordon McFadzean
Mr & Mrs John McKenzie
Mr Neil McMaster
Miss C. McCleod
Mr & Mrs Warren Moore
Miss C. A. Pearse
Mrs E. Pearse
Mr Nigel Pool
Dr & Mrs H. F. Pile
Mr & Mrs Harry Penman
Rev Michael Perry
Mr Rodney Picot
Mrs Eunice Pinniger
Mr Keith Richardson
Mr C. Rose
Mr & Mrs Gerald Riley
Mr Ian Rolson
Mr & Mrs Philip Restall
Mr & Mrs John Sibley

Mr Nigel Skinner
Mr Andrew Sneller
Mr & Mrs Mike Smith
Miss Dawn Shaw
Miss Bridget Simpson
Miss Emily Shaw
Mrs V. Stockman
Mr M. Thomas
Miss N. Tyler
Mr Ken Trenchard
Dr & Mrs Roland Travis
Miss Sarah Tozer
Mr & Mrs Wadsworth
Mr M. Waterson
Mr & Mrs J. G. Williams
Mr J. Workman
Mrs A. Wagstaff
Mr Glen Winder
Mr & Mrs Ron Walker
Mrs S. Wade
Mr & Mrs David Wetton
Miss Mabel Wilson

Churches

All Saints, Brixham
Barclay Church, Edinburgh
Bushey Baptist Church
Bromsgrove Methodist Church
Brownhills West Methodist Church
Brownhills Methodist
Barlaston Methodist
Churches of Chalke Valley, West Salisbury (the hover-garage)
Church of Scotland and Free Churches of the Royal Air Force
Clayhanger Methodist
Ebbesbourne Wake Women's Fellowship
Gorsley Baptist
Glanrafon Evangelical Church
Great Wyrley Methodist
Hirwaun Eng Methodist
Harnham Free Church
Kendall Road Baptist
Long Port Methodist
Leeds University Methodist Chaplaincy
Lawnton Baptist Church (Queensland)
Lenzie Union Parish
Norton Canes Methodist
Penkridge Methodist
Pelsall Methodist
The *Methodist Recorder*
Retford Baptist
St Andrews, Finningley

St Barnabas, Cambridge
St John's, Woodbridge
St Mary's, Brixham
St Mary's, Wirral
St Paul's, Jersey
St Saviour's, Guildford
Stoke Holy Cross
Send Evangelical Church
Spring Hill Methodist
Sheffield Methodist
Tisbury Fellowship
Tisbury Methodist
Tonbridge Parish
Woodbridge Methodist
Walsall Wood Methodist

Commercial Supporters
Andrew Weir Shipping Ltd, Bank Line
AAlco Air Solent Ltd
Air Niugini
British Telecom Laboratories Ltd
British Petroleum - Papua New Guinea Pty
BP service station, Mosman, Australia
Bowring Aviation Ltd
Kila Bowring, PNG
Clarks Active Air Shoes
Clarke's Industrial Agencies
Century Group of Companies Pty
Crewsaver Ltd
EMT - PNG Television
Ewevale Printing Publishers Ltd
Forestart Ltd
Fuji Films Ltd
GEC, Marconi Dynamics Ltd
GEC, Marconi Defence Systems Ltd
Herbert Pool Ltd
Hi-Lift Services Port Moresby
Hobden Davis Ltd
Ok Tedi Mining Co
Optyl (Australia) Pty
P & O European Ferries Ltd
R. Perry & Co Ltd
Laurabada Shipping Services Pty Ltd
Legal & General Insurance Co Ltd
B. C. Leather Pty
Maxell UK Ltd
Mitchell North West Ltd
J. P. Morgan (Australia)
Mark 1 Agencies
Pine River Locksmith
Premier Warehousing Ltd

Royal Bank of Scotland, Holts Branch
Saracen Fire West Gloucester
Shell Papua New Guinea Pty
Singapore Airlines
Square Two Badge Co
Snia (UK) Ltd
Thurston Avionics Ltd

Pharmaceutical Supporters

Astra Pharmaceuticals Ltd
Abbott Laboratories Ltd
Allen & Hanbury's Ltd
Beecham Research
Echo (Joint Mission Hospital Equipment Board Ltd)
Glaxo Laboratories Ltd
Fisons Ltd
Lilly Industries Ltd
Merck Sharp & Dohme Ltd
Parke-Davis Ltd
Rousseu Ltd
Smith Kline & Beecham Pharmaceuticals
The Wellcome Foundation

Support from Official Organisations

British High Commission, Port Moresby
Southampton Community Hospital Services
Royal Air Force
Royal Australian Air Force
The Services and Sound Vision Corporation

Charitable Trusts

The Beatrice Laing Trust

Appendix D
Medical Report of the PNG Hovercraft Expedition

The Team

Dr Bill Gould and Dr Rachel Pinniger planned and supervised the medical programme. Miss Aileen Boyd and Miss Sarah Williams joined the team as part of the elective period of their final year of medical studies at the universities of Edinburgh and Cambridge respectively. We benefited by the recruitment to the team of a flight-lieutenant seconded from the Royal Australian Air Force, Dr Rachel Grimmer, who quickly integrated into the team.

Aims and Objectives

1. To ensure the whole hovercraft team were adequately prepared medically for the expedition.
2. To ensure the team remained healthy throughout the expedition and received appropriate treatment in case of illness or accident.
3. To prepare adequate medical and surgical supplies for the team.
4. To attract donations of medicines and equipment for use at Balimo Health Centre.
5. To assist in the total medical programme of Balimo Health Centre both in the hospital and in the outreach programme as required.
6. To teach and provide adequate experience for the medical

students in the team.
7. To observe and to learn from the health care system of the PNG government.

Preparation
Eight months prior to the expedition we circulated each team member with the following.

1. A questionnaire to screen for potential medical problems and to obtain general information such as age, sex and family profile.

2. Advice about necessary immunisations (polio, tetanus, typhoid, hepatitis A, hepatitis B, BCG); malaria prophylaxis (chloroquine 2 tabs weekly plus maloprim 1 tab weekly); the avoidance of mosquito bites by using mosquito nets, insect repellent and suitable clothing; and the importance of drinking only safe water (either boiled or filtered). Each team member was advised to purchase their own personal water purifier.

3. A request to ascertain their own blood group. Every team member signed a document in which they acknowledged there were inherent dangers in going on the expedition, and accepted full financial responsibility for any illness, disability and death that might result from any pre-existing medical condition. They also promised to insure themselves and to accept full responsibility for any necessary medical care and the cost of repatriation. In the event of death, injury, illness or incapacity they promised that neither they nor anyone on their behalf would assert any claim or make any demand against the expedition or any member of it.

In our research for the best medical insurance we concluded

that both WEXAS and Endsleigh offered adequate cover. Three months before leaving for PNG we circulated a simple fitness programme to each team member, based on the Canadian Air Force Fitness programme.

The Health Services of Papua New Guinea

Health work in Papua New Guinea was begun by missionaries and government patrol officers. Both services have continued running in parallel until the present.

The churches provide 80 per cent of health work in the rural sector, and overall about 50 per cent. Some churches have also become involved in providing tertiary health services as well. Funding of the churches' health services comes from grants in aid from the government which in some cases can be 100 per cent of all running costs. Basic drugs and equipment are supplied by the government.

The present health system in PNG is based on recommendations from WHO. It aims to provide a health facility within three hours' walk of everyone in the country. The facilities provided range from base hospitals with national regional and provincial services down through provincial hospitals, district hospitals, health centres, health sub-centres and aid posts.

The base hospitals are staffed with specialists such as pathologists, radiologists, oncologists. Provincial hospitals have specialist surgeons, physicians, paediatricians and obstetricians. District hospitals usually have one doctor, while health centres are staffed by a health extension officer (HEO). Health sub-centres have only nurses, and aid posts have community health workers. Papua New Guinea was one of the first countries in the developing world to plan the distribution of its health services throughout the urban and rural sectors.

Training of health workers below the grade of medical practitioner has been largely set in rural areas so that the practical experience has been appropriate and workers thus trained have been more likely to stay working in those areas.

Due to the lack of doctors it falls to registered nurses and HEOs to do much of the admitting, diagnosing and prescribing for patients.

Doctors tend to have a more supervisory and teaching role than they do in Western countries. This graded approach to the delivery of health care where primary and some secondary care is administered by health workers other than doctors has been very effective and is a model which has been adapted by other countries. The relative success of the PNG model is due to three factors:

1. Standard treatment protocols in paediatrics, medicine and obstetrics.

2. A standard list of drugs and equipment graded for each level of the service.

3. Built-in arrangements for supervision and assessment. This important function is tending to be neglected in many areas.

The Balimo Health Centre

This unit started as an aid post after World War II and was staffed by a government first aid worker. Since 1966 it has been handed over to the Evangelical Church of Papua New Guinea and is now part of the Church Health Services of PNG. The ECP runs it under a contract agreement with the Provincial and National Health departments. The land it stands on its government-owned but almost all the buildings and equipment have been provided by the church.

The practice population is about 25,000 but its specialist surgical service extends to about 100,000 in the Western Province. Although called a health centre, it is in fact normally staffed with three doctors, one of whom is a specialist surgeon. It tends to attract medical, obstetric and surgical referrals from a wider area and thus functions more as a provincial hospital. The reason for its build-up in size and services far beyond the size of a health centre has been due to its being the teaching hospital for the Balimo School of Nursing which is currently training registered general nurses. The surgical programme at Balimo was a necessary adjunct of the nurse training school and was required by the PNG Nursing Council in 1985.

The health work by the church at Balimo is committed to the training of Christian registered nurses; an appropriate level of secondary health care; high-quality primary health care and the development, disciplining and discipling of its staff. Currently the health centre employs 70 people and has about 120 beds.

The Balimo Health Centre staffs and supervises six (6) large health sub-centres and fourteen aid posts. The HSCs each have a few obstetric and general beds and all have access to Balimo by two-way radio. Patients can be transferred by boat or aeroplane. All the local villages are visited by the Maternal Child Health clinic team monthly and the more distant villages are visited every three months. The clinics include Bible teaching, health education, family planning, ante-natal care and nutritional advice. Immunisation is given for tuberculosis, measles, whooping cough, tetanus, diphtheria and poliomyelitis. Leprosy cases are supervised and all primary and secondary schoolchildren get dental care. Houses, sanitation and water supplies are inspected. In-service courses are held for all staff as often as funding will allow.

The Role of the Medical Team

We were warmly welcomed by the staff at Balimo and invited to help in the outpatient department, wards and operating theatres etc. We were also able to accompany the community health team on their visits to villages for MCH clinics and school health checks. Most of these were done by dugout canoe but on occasion the doctors become flying doctors, going to health sub-centres by MAF planes. Some of these trips will be done later by hovercraft.

Our role in looking after the hovercraft team was primarily in giving advice on minor ailments and to remind the team that Sunday was malaria tablet day. Wonderfully, there was no serious illness and no accident to any team member — our prayers were answered!

The medical students certainly benefited from their exposure to Third World medicine and were able to see malaria and TB cases in abundance — major problems in PNG. They had a fair spectrum of exotica with crocodile bites, snakebites (PNG has the world's most poisonous snakes), patients gored by pigs and shot by arrows whilst out hunting, and patients suffering from a condition perhaps peculiar to this part of the world, an acute, sometimes fatal, haemolytic anaemia caused by eating sago (their staple diet) that is more than three weeks old.

The primary aim of the expedition was to strengthen the existing transportation system on the rivers and lagoons for patient care and health care delivery by using hovercraft in addition to canoes and planes.

We trust we have laid the foundations of the hoverdoctor service in the Western Province of PNG so that even more lives can be saved through the work of the Balimo Health Centre. Though our help seemed to be appreciated, in fact we learned much in our time at Balimo and returned home much richer and wiser for the experience.

W. M. Gould, MB ChB FRCS DTM & H
R. G. Pinniger, MB ChB MRCP DCH DRCOG (Obst) DTM & H